Knowing One's Medical Fate in Advance

Challenges for Diagnosis and Treatment, Philosophy, Ethics and Religion

Editors

Georg Pfleiderer Basel

Manuel Battegay Basel

Klaus Lindpaintner Newark, Del.

4 figures, 2 in color, 2012

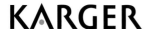 Basel · Freiburg · Paris · London · New York · New Delhi · Bangkok ·
Beijing · Tokyo · Kuala Lumpur · Singapore · Sydney

Prof. Dr. Georg Pfleiderer
Faculty of Theology
University of Basel
Missionsstrasse 17a
CH–4055 Basel
Switzerland

Prof. Dr. Manuel Battegay
Division of Infectious Diseases and
Hospital Epidemiology
University Hospital Basel
Petersgraben 4
CH–4031 Basel
Switzerland

Prof. Dr. Klaus Lindpaintner
SDIX
111 Pencader Drive
Newark, DE 19702
USA

This book was generously supported by the 'Freiwillige Akademische Gesellschaft', and the 'Schweizerische Akademie der Medizinischen Wissenschaften (SAMW)'

SAMW
Schweizerische Akademie
der Medizinischen
Wissenschaften

ASSM
Académie Suisse
des Sciences Médicales

ASSM
Accademia Svizzera delle
Scienze Mediche

SAMS
Swiss Academy
of Medical Sciences

Library of Congress Cataloging-in-Publication Data

Knowing one's medical fate in advance : challenges for diagnosis and
treatment, philosophy, ethics and religion/ editors, Georg Pfleiderer,
Manuel Battegay, Klaus Lindpaintner.
     p. ; cm.
  Includes bibliographical references and index.
  ISBN 978-3-8055-9649-7 (hard cover : alk. paper) -- ISBN 978-3-8055-9650-3
(e-ISBN)
  I. Pfleiderer, Georg. II. Battegay, Manuel. III. Lindpaintner, Klaus.
  [DNLM: 1. Patients--psychology. 2. Prognosis. 3. Genetic Predisposition
to Disease--psychology. 4. Religion and Medicine. 5. Truth Disclosure. W
85]

  616.07'5--dc23

                                                2012007745

Bibliographic Indices. This publication is listed in bibliographic services, including Current Contents® and Index Medicus.

© Copyright 2012 by S. Karger AG, P.O. Box, CH–4009 Basel (Switzerland)
www.karger.com
Printed in Germany on acid-free and non-aging paper (ISO 9706) by Kraft Druck GmbH, Ettlingen
ISBN 978-3-8055-9649-7
e-ISBN 978-3-8055-9650-3

Contents

Pfleiderer G, Battegay M, Lindpaintner K (eds): Knowing One's Medical Fate in Advance. Challenges for Diagnosis and Treatment, Philosophy, Ethics and Religion. Basel, Karger, 2012, pp 1–5

Introduction

Modern medicine is increasingly bringing the future to the present. Novel diagnostic procedures allow advanced medical prognoses quantifying the future outcome of an illness and its course. Thus, the understanding of the likelihood of therapeutic strategies to succeed or fail in an individual patient is becoming ever more transparent. Individuals are facing the complicated task of transferring these risk assessments to fit their personal life perspectives, develop anticipatory 'coping strategies', and, quite often, make concrete decisions and choices about themselves.

How does a person feel when faced with a 20% risk of contracting cancer of the intestine in the next 10–15 years? How do expectant parents deal with a 1:280 chance of having a child with trisomy 21? What are the criteria for responsible decisions in such situations? – Increasing prognostic accuracy of modern medicine, paradoxically, brings about a new dimension of uncertainty for the individual, whether still healthy or already a patient. Prognoses may evolve due to on-going progress in medical research. Examples are the constantly evolving arsenal of new anti-cancer medications, or the fundamental progress seen in treating infectious diseases such as HIV. Questions thus arising with regard to medical ethics are often vexing as an ever-increasing understanding of one's own medical fate goes hand in hand with continued uncertainty and lack of knowledge. This concerns both the individuals with a certain prognosis and their relatives as well as the medical experts who are called upon to provide advice and council patients and their relatives. Converting a medical prognosis into a subjective understanding and reassessment of life quality may pose existential difficulties.

New-found prognostic technologies may also affect prenatal life. Owing to progress in genetic testing, the possibility of recognizing prenatal health risks before physical signs of disease are visible is now possible. This presents the individual with a plethora of new challenges. Improved ability of looking into the future now allows us to not only prognosticate the course of a disease, but to actually predict future health problems long before any signs or symptoms are apparent.

The future implications of these developments for society, especially of predictive genetic testing, have recently become the focus of active investigation. The challenge of anticipation of one's future medical problems raises a multitude of fundamental and difficult ethical questions. What answers can specialized modern medical ethics and practical philosophy provide? What legal questions must be considered? And how can the paradigm-shift presented by modern medical diagnostics be integrated into historical and cultural frameworks?

Many people are touched by the religious dimension of their lives. What answers can religion and theology provide to help coping with the prospect of a future about which we know increasingly more, but still remains uncertain? Anticipation of the future is dealt with in many ways by religion, e.g. in the prophesy and hope of the kingdom of God. Can religion provide coping strategies to help overcome the life crises brought about by a medical prognosis, or a predictive test?

The volume at hand is based on a conference convened in Basel in June 2010, organized by Karger Publishers under the auspices of the University of Basel and chaired by the signatories. It was the goal of the conference to bring together specialists from diverse fields of medicine, ethics, philosophy, religious science and theology. The aim was to encourage wide-ranging discussion among a broad audience to generate ideas and approaches towards tackling the implications of the new 'knowledge of the future' on societal and individual ethical values. As part of the conference, a workshop organized by Dr. Theol. Gabriella Brahier gave young scientists the opportunity to present their own research on the topic and to share it with distinguished experts. There was also a MA seminar connected with the conference at the Theological Faculty held during the spring semester.

The volume contains most of the papers given at the conference in revised versions. The book also provides transcripts/summaries of the question-and-answer sessions following the presentation of each paper (with the exception of the paper by A. Brueninghaus and R. Porz).

The volume is divided into three sections: 'Medical Perspectives', 'Ethical and Juridical Perspectives' and 'Religious Perspectives'.

The first section, 'Medical Perspectives', is introduced by the physician-scientist Manuel Battegay. Battegay demonstrates as one example of an impressive success story in medicine the dramatic improvements witnessed over the last 15 years in the therapy and prognosis of HIV infection. The advances give impressive proof that prognosis can change in a very short time period and knowing one's medical fate might be difficult – from the physicians and patients perspective.

Among the most complex challenges for medical professionals as well as for patients concerned might be the knowledge about medical conditions that affect the personal ability of 'knowing', i.e. of intellectual function, such as presented by diseases like Alzheimer's dementia. The neuroscientist, Andreas Papassotiropoulos, shows that a tremendous gap remains between prognostic statements based on genetic research and the actual fate of an individual or the quality of his/her memory. Despite a growing market of products offering gene test-based 'personalized medicine', the actual predictive power of such tests for the individual is usually negligible.

Another emerging field to which genetic testing is applied as a predictive tool – resulting in complex challenges for individual ethical decision making – is prenatal diagnostics. The volume's second section, 'Ethical and Juridical Perspectives', thus begins with an article on this topic by the bioethicist and protestant theologian, Gabriella Brahier. Based on qualitative interviews with consenting pregnant women she analyses individual processes of ethical decision-making. She concludes that these processes are – appropriately – guided by the ethical concept of biographical authenticity. She argues that insights thus derived may modify abstract models of 'informed consent' and provide reason for a more proactive and interactive view of the physician's role in the process of prenatal consultation.

Huntington's chorea is a rare hereditary monogenic disease. Owing to the highly predictive power of testing for the disease in affected families, it serves as a paradigmatic example of issues surrounding the topic of prediction of future health events. This results in important psychological, sometimes existential, challenges for the person who may want to be tested; it also impacts close relatives (sons/daughters, and even more so parents) in diverse ways, including questions related to family planning. In their joint article, Anne Brünighaus (social education theory) and Rouven Porz (philosophy) shed light on the often conflictual decision-making processes associated with such a test as well as the coping strategies that help individuals deal with the ambiguity of attaining such knowledge. Consideration of coping strategies must take into account that both the decision to know and the decision not to know intimately affects others, namely the decision-maker's relatives.

These examples highlight how gene technology, or at least certain aspects of it, present an entirely new type of predictive information about our future and confront us with new requirements of dealing with this knowledge. Does this possibly even fundamentally affect our image of man ('Menschenbild')? The philosopher and ethicist, Dieter Birnbaum, argues that in a general and descriptive sense that this is not the case; it may, however, change the way the individual deals with his/her personal (predicted) future. This, in turn, may affect our perception of medical ethics: Does patient autonomy as a moral right imply a right to know in the sense that the physician is obliged to give the patient all the information he/she has access to? If interpreted exclusively as a 'presumed consent' (i.e. 'opting out') autonomy principle, withholding (partial) information of his/her prospective future from an individual would be ethically wrong only if it was against the patient's (presumed or outspoken) will. In addition, considerations such as the avoidance of serious harm for the patient may occasionally argue for disclosing or withholding information. The way information is provided should always be adjusted to the ability of the individual to control his/her autonomy.

A related topic is the legal implications surrounding the disclosure of predictive medical information. Bianca Doerr, a legal scholar, reflects on the Swiss Federal Act on Genetic Testing in Humans (HGTA) and its intention to balance the ethical principles of autonomy and beneficence regarding the disclosure of genetic information. While the basic principle of autonomy postulates the right of self-determination of the individual (specifically with regard to the right to know and the right not to know), there is one particular limitation of this right: in the case of 'overriding interests' of certain other individuals, particularly close relatives, an individual's genetic information can be disclosed even without his/her consent. Executing this provision, of course, is a very difficult task requiring deep judicial, medical and ethical reflection.

Making decisions in the face of these ambiguities will often challenge some of the most fundamental beliefs of the individuals concerned. These may often, albeit certainly not always, relate to their religious faith. Addressing this, three selected perspectives from diverse fields of religious bioethics are presented in this volume's third section, 'Religious Perspectives'.

Benjamin Gesundheit, physician and ethicist, points out that Jewish medical ethics has always endorsed diverse and differentiated views. Nevertheless, there has always been consensus among Jewish scholars that, if at all possible, medical healing should be attempted and a passively fatalistic attitude should be avoided.

In contrast to pagan fatalism, the belief in divine providence regarding the future of individuals' lives has always been a principal element of Christianity, as the Protestant theologian and ethicist, Georg Pfleiderer, points out. Christian theology is always suspended in the tension between justification taking place in the past or the future and the immanent or transcendent fulfillment of life. Twentieth century Protestant theology emphasizes the former. Thus, it is guided by an attitude of calmness and ease in dealing with the challenges that predictive medicine, and in particular genetic testing, may hold for us as individuals.

How do Asian religions, namely Buddhism, conceptualize the ethical problems of predictive medicine? The religious scholar, Jens Schlieter, expands on a philosophical understanding of religion as a coping mechanism for the finality of our existence. Thus, in dealing with the terminal stages of an illness it may be helpful to imply the concept of a 'point of no return', where medical intervention should be replaced by palliative approaches. From a religious perspective, this concept is aligned with the distinction between the healing and rescuing aspects of belief. This interpretative model is useful to understand the Buddhist concept of karma and its role in dealing with illness. Karma must neither be understood as a single-cause explanation of disease as the consequence of sin, nor is it based on a sharp distinction between immanence and transcendence. Rather, it represents an attempt of finding a balance between contingency and destiny from one's own perspective. Viewed from the perspective of karma, one's medical future cannot be known; nevertheless it becomes present when one's life-span is exhausted. At that point of no return the primacy of healing must yield to the primacy of rescue, 'because he or she already belongs, in part, to another realm'.

As editors of this volume, we would like to thank all our colleagues from diverse disciplines who presented papers at the conference, participated in discussions and/ or made contributions to this volume. We also wish to express our gratitude to Karger Publishers, namely to Mrs. Gabriella and Dr. Thomas Karger, for their generous support which made the conference and this publication possible.

For significant financial support of the conference and this publication, we wish to acknowledge the Freiwillige Akademische Gesellschaft Basel (FAG) and the Schweizerische Akademie der Medizinischen Wissenschaften (SAMW).

Georg Pfleiderer, Manuel Battegay, Klaus Lindpaintner
Basel, 2012

Medical Perspectives

Pfleiderer G, Battegay M, Lindpaintner K (eds): Knowing One's Medical Fate in Advance. Challenges for Diagnosis and Treatment, Philosophy, Ethics and Religion. Basel, Karger, 2012, pp 6–14

Evolving Therapy and Prognosis in HIV – How Knowing One's Medical Fate in Advance Can Change Dramatically

Manuel Battegay

Division of Infectious Diseases & Hospital Epidemiology, University Hospital Basel, Basel, Switzerland

To know one's medical fate in advance is difficult if not impossible even if, as with the human immunodeficiency virus/acquired immune deficiency syndrome (HIV/ AIDS), a very serious prognosis seemed clear just some years ago. Specific parameters and factors of a specific disease may be stable enabling a quite precise prognosis, however, there is still a high degree of uncertainty, also with all the knowledge we have. In this presentation I will show how things can evolve very, very quickly and that prognosis 15 years ago was not the same as it is now, especially with HIV/AIDS.

The change of perspective can be observed with Time Magazine covers. In the early years a disease with unknown origin was first described: what is AIDS, what is HIV? In 1983, the important discovery of the virus for which the Nobel prize was given to Barré Sinoussi and Luc Montaigner in 2008 was made. Time magazine well representing the general atmosphere gave bad news: 'The Growing Threat', 'The Big Chill', 'Losing the Battle'. This was just 15 years ago. In 1996, research on the viral replication gave a perspective on modern treatments which were introduced with much hope at that time.

After infection the virus disseminates and causes already after few days an important immune damage. Nevertheless, the immune defense eventually combats the virus leading usually to a significant decrease of viremia, i.e. the concentration of the virus in the blood. Afterwards the immune function decreases as measured by an excellent surrogate marker, i.e. the CD4-T cell lymphocytes [1]. The risk of opportunistic infections or tumors increases then due to impaired cellular immunity.

Prognosis and Advances in Treatment

When a patient achieved severe immune deficiency, i.e. a CD4-T cell level below 200 cells/μl, survival was rare beyond two year as there were no good treatment options available.

A landmark study published in 1997 showed that by measuring HIV viral load and CD4-T cells the probability to have AIDS, i.e. the disease, within 3 years could be predicted [1]. For example, a patient with high viral load above 100'000 copies/mL and low CD4-T cell counts had a very severe prognosis as stated above. One has to keep in mind that this was only 13 years ago and that today such a patient with treatment has a completely different prognosis.

What happened between 1996 and today was unexpected and unprecedent – the progress of HIV treatment was fabulous. In the late eighties HIV drugs were not effective beyond six months of therapy. From 1996 on several new HIV drugs were used in combination, showing a dramatic reduction in morbidity and mortality [2]. Briefly, the mechanism for treatment works via stopping the replication cycle of HIV at very different stages of the virus/cell cycle. In particular, drugs stopping the activity of the HIV reverse transcriptase and protease are most effective and inhibit the virus copy machine with a frequency of 10 billion times a day very efficiently.

Treatment Goals, Cautious Prognosis, and Perceptions

The goals of antiretroviral therapy are a sustained suppression of the HIV replication, the regeneration of CD4-T cells, an improvement in immune system function and thereby the reduction in opportunistic infections and tumors. The Swiss HIV Cohort Study described the significant increase of CD4-T cells under treatment in the first large observational study with over 5,000 patients with a significant impact on prognosis. The study of Egger et al. [2] shows the change in outcome and prognosis with new combination treatments. The proportion of patients who survived increased from 10% to 70% [2]. An updated analysis shows that prognosis was even better in the years to come (Figure 1). This change in outcome is due, as pathophysiological studies showed later on, not only to an increase in numbers of CD4-T cells but also in an increase in the function of immune cells which can again combat pathogens responsible for opportunistic diseases.

As one can imagine the change of prognosis in the late nineties led to a very positive reaction if not euphoria first by scientists and physicians followed later when trust in therapies was built up also in patients.

Knowing one's medical fate in advance – in that time as a doctor one had to be very cautious with statements about prognosis. In this context it is important to mention that even in view of the excellent prognosis of nowadays HIV treatments a patient may go through different phases of perception regarding his disease as explained below. Vice versa the perception of doctors is important too and essential to initiate

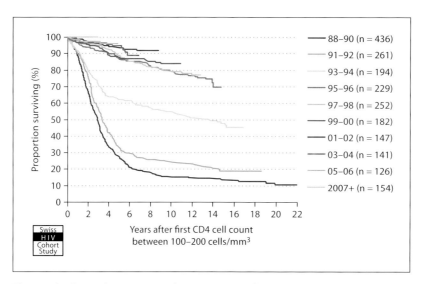

Fig. 1. The figure demonstrates the proportion of patients surviving in different time periods after the first CD4-T cell count has been measured between 100–200 cells/µl. Note that only a few patients survived in the early years (1988–1990), whereas over 90% of patients survive in recent years. Figure courtesy of Matthias Egger, University of Bern, Switzerland.

treatment. For example, a large study of the Swiss HIV Cohort Study could demonstrate that treatment was withheld for some intravenous drug users [3]. The perception at that time was that the treatment was too complicated for this group of patients and would therefore be not successful. We might say that knowing the others fate in advance should be also always viewed critically and adapted if wrong.

Perception Models

There are well-established models of awareness by Prochaska et al. on behavioral research [4] that describe the stages of change: precontemplation, contemplation, preparation, action, and maintenance. We used a simplified version of the available models for HIV [5, 6] and presented this information in one table to help physicians, nurses, and patients.

For example, in 'precontemplation' a patient might say, 'I will survive without treatment', 'I don't need it, I feel good', or 'I don't want to think about it'. But with lower CD4 T cells, he/she might contemplate treatment. It is most important to discuss data with a patient possibly changing the perception caused by wrong or insufficient information (www.europeanaidsclinicalsociety.org).

'Preparation' marks the stage when the patient says, 'I want to start, I think the drugs will help me live a normal life'. Usually, this is the stage just before initiation of treatment. As stated above prognosis changed dramatically. From 2006 on it became obvious that the prognosis between HIV-positive patients and a HIV-negative normal population did not differ strongly anymore, at least in a large part [7]. However, survival still depends on individual factors such as illicit drug use, co-infections with the hepatitis viruses B and C or other conditions. The strongest individual factor for prognosis is associated again with behavior, i.e. adherence and continuous therapy [8, 9]. Many studies indicate that an insufficient level of drug intake has severe sequelae on resistance development, treatment effect and consequently survival.

'Wunderbar' – 'Wonderful'

These were the words of a patient entering the consultation room 2006. This patient was 43 years old, HIV-infected in 1987 and also diagnosed with chronic hepatitis C. HIV responded successfully to antiretroviral treatment. The viral load was since treatment start 10 years ago undetectable and the immune system close to normal. How did perception from a deadly disease change so strongly? Well, he married 3 years ago, his wife is HIV-negative and the couple has a healthy HIV-negative child.

Continuing Developments

Is the picture too rosy, is there an important aspect missing for knowing one's medical fate in advance? Yes – as many drugs demonstrate mild but sometimes also severe side effects. However, it is difficult to precisely predict if a specific side effect will affect a specific individual. Nevertheless, progress has been done also in this field. E.g., one drug (abacavir) may lead to severe hypersensitivity in 5% of individuals. Today we can highly predict whether the likelihood of this hypersensitivity reaction is extremely low, i.e. close to 0% or whether it is approximately 50%. It this context the abacavir related hypersensitivity only occurs in HLA B5701 positive individuals, allowing to anticipate this potential life-threatening side effect in predisposed patients.

In conclusion the treatment development is still ongoing and as figure 1 demonstrates we assume that life prolongation is bringing many individuals to a close to normal life expectancy. The change of treatment success had consequences on guidelines and concepts of treatment as shown in figure 2. In 1996, in the upcoming of combination antiretroviral treatment, there were still hopes that the virus could be eradicated. Hence, all patients were treated. Thereafter, when it became clear that this is not possible an early start was recommended to preserve immunity. Afterwards more pessimistic views prevailed becoming aware of the long-term toxicity and co-morbidities of the first line drugs. Following this, the start of treatment was delayed. With better treatments the threshold to initiate treatment earlier decreased. Now treatment concepts change again as it becomes obvious that

1996	Hit hard, hit early	Hope of cure
	CD4	
1997	<500	Conservation of immunity
2000	<350	ART works at lower levels
2003	<200	ART long-term toxicity
2007	<350	Reduce morbidity, less toxicity
2008	<350	Comorbidity (non-AIDS), readiness
2010	or higher	Remaining morbidity
2011?	All?	Comorbidity, readiness, transmisssion(?)

Fig. 2. This table shows different treatment concepts changing from hope of cure to less optimistic treatment goals. The lower threshold of CD4-T cells depicts a lower degree of immunity. For example, in 2003 treatment was started only late in disease course to prevent long-term toxicity and enable a patient as long as possible to live without treatment. However, with better treatments which are much better tolerable the threshold of CD4-T cells increased, i.e. combination antiretroviral treatment is started much earlier to reduce the remaining morbidity.

transmission is significantly reduced with successful combination antiretroviral therapy. Hence, the question is whether to treat all patients as in the mid nineties, but with a different concept.

'I Will Survive this Challenge'

What are the challenges nowadays? This is best illustrated by a patient history. A patient came with these words: 'Ich werde auch diese Herausforderung überleben' – 'I will survive also this challenge'. This 46-year-old patient was HIV-infected since 1994 with advanced stage disease. He started therapy in 1999. In 2003, he suffered from acute hepatitis C, which was cured with interferon therapy without any recurrence. In 2005, he was diagnosed with a diffuse tumor of the colon and it was then when he said that he will survive also this third life threatening challenge. He was successfully operated and treated. Since then he is asymptomtic, fully working, without any recurrence.

Prognosis Outside of Europe

In other countries circumstances are different – there is a dramatic global pandemia with over 30 million infected people. Patients present to care more often late or too

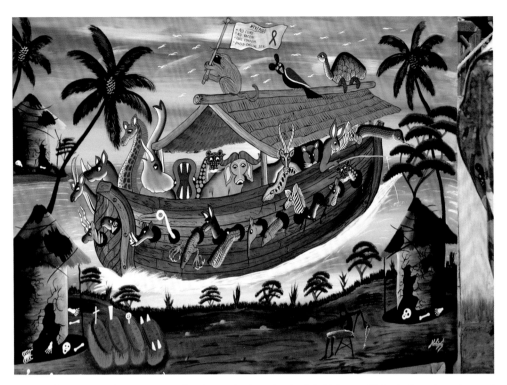

Fig. 3. This picture demonstrates the dramatic situation in Sub-Saharan Africa before the advent of antiretrovirals: in most parts with no cure, no vaccine, use condom, avoid casual sex as inscribed on the flag. Figure courtesy of Marcel Stoeckle, University of Basel, Switzerland. The artist lived in Dar-es-Salaam, Tanzania and died from AIDS.

late, in particular in Sub-Saharan Africa and Eastern Europe. Many of newly infected people outside of developed countries are unaware to the possibilities of modern medicine and, thus, their perception is really pessimistic. This is shown by the artful expression of an Noah' Ark (figure 3). Importantly, in many regions, in particular rural areas, treatment possibilities and access to health care system are lacking or still insufficient. However, treatment possibilities are also increasing in Africa and now 6 million people are treated worldwide with the highest increase in Sub-Saharan Africa. This is illustrated by a project in the Kilombero valley of Tanzania supported by the Swiss Tropical- & Public Health Institute and the University Hospitals of Basel and Berne, Switzerland, where more than 5,000 HIV-infected patients are cared in a chronic diseases clinic. For survival aspects such healthcare facilities, the number of doctors and nutrition are essential factors influencing prognosis and the knowledge about one's own medical fate.

In summary, I hope I could demonstrate that knowing one's medical fate can be very relative on an individual but also epidemological level. Although the example of progress for HIV/AIDS diagnosis and treatment is probably unprecedent in such a short time span, uncertainty and lack of precision is much more the case than assumed by physicians and patients – simply we do not know ahead of time everything even if we are 'sure'.

Acknowledgement

The author is grateful to Dr. Luigia Elzi for critical review of the manuscript.

Questions and Answers

Q. [*Klaus Lindpaintner*]: There is a mutation in the CCR5 receptor, the delta 32 mutation, which is actually protective against a negative outcome of a HIV infection. How would you as a HIV physician feel if such a variation is present in a given patient?

A. [*Battegay*]: Usually if a patient is infected, the chance is very low that he has the actual mutation. Mostly, those patients who have the mutation are not infected. But you are right, some are infected and they have a better disease course. Additionally, there are other factors of the HLA, the transplantation antigen, which are associated with rapid or slow progression. We do not routinely measure such mutations but we hope to develop tests that we may use routinely to know in whom the disease will progress rapidly or slowly and to answer the question more precisely when to initiate treatment.

Q. [*Mr. Gyr, Basel*]: Are there populations that are less prone to become infected? For instance, in Bangladesh, they think that to be the case, but I don't know whether there is any proof yet?

A. [*Battegay*]: This is a very good point. One of the most important preventive factors is male circumcision. If men are circumcised, it is estimated that the risk of HIV transmission is reduced by 60%. One theory is that in populations and societies where the percentage of circumcision is extremely high there is an effect on the population level for HIV transmission.

For example in Zanzibar, the percentage of HIV-infected people is below 1%, but in mainland Tanzania, it is around 5%. This is a very significant difference which may be due to the differences in male circumcision habits. Hence, people in Bangladesh might really be less prone to infection.

Q. [*Mark Schweda*]: One aspect of knowing one's medical fate in advance in connection with HIV and AIDS in the 1980s and 1990s was by taking the HIV test. I remember a lot of people back then saying, they would not even want to take the test, or some took the test and would not collect their results. What is your experience? Or are there even any figures on how the development of therapies has influenced people's attitudes towards taking the test?

A. [*Battegay*]: Again this is a very important aspect, and there is a tremendous change in many ways. In Western countries, the HIV test has become almost routine and the attitude towards it is more 'relaxed'. Knowing that one is HIV-infected is very important as there are very good treatments available, and also in order to prevent transmission of the disease to others. As stated, transmission can be reduced by effective treatments. In Africa, awareness has changed immensely and the test frequency has increased sharply since treatments have become available. Before that, HIV testing was not performed as there was no hope of treatment. Secondly, there is pressure urging for the tests to be carried out more often so that a more precise prevention program can be initiated. Basically, we go back to the principles of infectious diseases. Prevention works primarily if you go to the people who are already infected. This is a basic principle, because, if you try to use prevention all over, people get disinterested or are not convinced. It is observed now throughout Africa that voluntary counseling and testing went up sharply especially in the vicinity of treatment clinics. This is a very strong argument for having the programs installed in many places. Many people in Africa are willing to take on the responsibility of prevention and treatment programs. The main challenges will be at the operational level with difficult circumstances in everyday life.

Q. [*Georg Pfleiderer*]: Can you perhaps say something more about this so-called subjective factor? How do people deal with it? There are huge numbers of people living with HIV today, in a sort postsymptomatic or asymptomatic condition. Could you tell us something about the strategies of dealing with this situation? Is getting the diagnosis still the most important moment in their life? Or has that also changed? Is it still a central element of their personal identity to be an HIV-positive person?

A. [*Battegay*]: First, I think it is important not to generalize and it is difficult to really know ahead what a patient will perceive. Some patients say they take the drugs in the morning and don't think about it at all for one moment before or afterwards. It lies beside their toothpaste and that's it. Obviously, they continue to function in life as they had done before. HIV has become routine.

For most patients though, I feel it is still a burden. It affects a central place in their life: their relationships and their sexuality. Also, it is a lifelong disease with lifelong treatment. Mostly, after the first phase, persons have adapted fairly well. They inform close friends and family and they experience that life can go on quite normally. What has brought about a huge difference is the possibility for couples to have children. Also an issue is convincing their friends and family that they will not necessarily die. This often takes some time. Although patients themselves feel very good, it takes a while until their families stop asking them all the time, 'how are you?', 'how do you feel?'. Hence, there is a whole variety of reactions, and yes, certainly, there are the dramatic moments in the beginning that prevail, but thereafter a lot of the trust comes back.

References

1 Mellors JW, Munoz A, Giorgi JV, et al: Plasma viral load and CD4+ lymphocytes as prognostic markers of HIV-1 infection. Ann Intern Med 1997;126:946–954.

2 Egger M, Hirschel B, Francioli P, et al: Impact of new antiretroviral combination therapies in HIV infected patients in Switzerland: prospective multicentre study. Swiss HIV Cohort Study. BMJ 1997; 315:1194–1199.

3 Bassetti S, Battegay M, Furrer H, et al: Why is highly active antiretroviral therapy (HAART) not prescribed or discontinued? Swiss HIV Cohort Study. J Acquir Immune Defic Syndr 1999;21:114–119.

4 Prochaska JO, DiClemente CC, Norcross JC: In search of how people change. Applications to addictive behaviors. Am Psychol 1992;47:1102–1114.

5 Willey C, Redding C, Stafford J, et al: Stages of change for adherence with medication regimens for chronic disease: development and validation of a measure. Clin Ther 2000;22:858–871.

6 Highstein GR, Willey C, Mundy LM: Development of Stage of Readiness and decisional balance instruments: tools to enhance clinical decision-making for adherence to antiretroviral therapy. AIDS Behav 2006;10:563–573.

7 Hogg R, Lima V, Sterne JA, et al: Life expectancy of individuals on combination antiretroviral therapy in high-income countries: a collaborative analysis of 14 cohort studies. Lancet 2008;372:293–299.

8 Glass TR, De Geest S, Hirschel B, et al: Self-reported non-adherence to antiretroviral therapy repeatedly assessed by two questions predicts treatment failure in virologically suppressed patients. Antivir Ther 2008;13:77–85.

9 Elzi L, Marzolini C, Furrer H, et al: Treatment modification in human immunodeficiency virus-infected individuals starting combination antiretroviral therapy between 2005 and 2008. Arch Intern Med 2010;170:57–65.

Prof. Dr. med. Manuel Battegay
Division of Infectious Diseases & Hospital Epidemiology
University Hospital Basel
Petersgraben 4
CH-4031 Basel (Switzerland)
Tel. +41 61 265 50 72, E-Mail mbattegay@uhbs.ch

Medical Perspectives

Pfleiderer G, Battegay M, Lindpaintner K (eds): Knowing One's Medical Fate in Advance. Challenges for Diagnosis and Treatment, Philosophy, Ethics and Religion. Basel, Karger, 2012, pp 15–25

Related to Human Cognition: Is Personalization Feasible and Desirable?

Andreas Papassotiropoulos

Division of Molecular Psychology, Life Sciences Training Facility, Biozentrum, University of Basel, Basel, Switzerland

When asked about genetics, many people think it is about prediction at the individual level, a kind of pre-determination, or in other words: 'knowing' for certain what is going to happen. The reality about human genetics is actually quite different. I will explain what genetics can do in the context of my discipline, what it cannot do, and perhaps, what it should not do. In my lecture I will focus on the science of molecular psychology, specifically on human memory.

I often am asked what psychology has to do with molecules. In fact, the right question would be: how is it possible that one could think psychology does not have anything to do with molecules? The organ which produces our emotions, thoughts, and cognition – is the brain. Of course, the brain and its functions are related to molecules.

I am not the only one to claim this. The giants have already thought of the idea of molecular psychology. For example, in 1859, Charles Darwin wrote in his *On the Origin of the Species*:

"In the distant future I see open fields for far more important researches. Psychology will be based on a new foundation, that of the necessary acquirement of each mental power and capacity by gradation."

Implying that psychology would be a far more important research than others, Charles Darwin imagined in 1859 that someday human genetics will contribute to the understanding of human mental power and capacity.

I address 5 important points about my view of human genetics, while keeping it as simple as possible:

1 Genetics of complex human traits and phenotypes is a tool to understand biology.
2 Genome-wide association studies revolutionize our knowledge on complex traits relevant to neuropsychiatry.

3   Genetic clusters rather than single genes are potential biomarkers.
4   The use of human genetic information will lead to improved characterization of complex human traits.
5   The combination of genetics with other relevant sources of information such as functional brain imaging (fMRI) will increase biological knowledge.

In neuroscience, we mostly study diseases or physiological traits that are complex. We have to understand and appreciate the need for multifactorial models: several genetic factors apply, but there is also the environment, comorbidity (the presence or absence of additional diseases), personality, sociodemographic factors, lifestyle, life events, and medication. Thus, there are several factors, each with a certain weight, which contributes to the development of a certain trait or disease.

What do we mean when talking about 'personalized medicine'? What do we want to do with 'personalized medicine' and how do we want to use human genetic information? Is it about prediction, whether one will develop a disease or not? Is it about diagnosis? Or is it pharmacogenomics? Irrespective of these issues, we have to realize this: human genetic information is related to probability. Furthermore, the way we want to use human genetic information does not only depend on probability but also on the consequences that this probability would have.

Let me give you an example related to Alzheimer's disease. This complex disease at its end stage is marked by severe atrophy of the hippocampus, a brain region related to memory. We believe that specific molecular events lead to the erroneous degradation of the amyloid precursor protein. In order to escape or break free from the metabolic pathway(s) leading to this disease, there are possibly several steps or stages, all of which are modified by genes. In other words, genes contribute to the direction that this metabolic cascade may take. Only if we could understand the nature and function of all contributing genes, we could know who is likely to develop this disease.

Some very rare cases of Alzheimer's disease are monogenic. For example, one of the first cases I saw when I was in Zürich was of a 32-year-old patient with full-blown Alzheimer's. From his family pedigree, it looked like a Mendelian segregation, specifically an autosomal dominant mode of inheritance. It is known that these rare cases are related to mutations in at least 3 genes: APP, PS-1, and PS-2. In his family, he had the PS-1 mutation.

If an individual has this PS-1 mutation, the probability of developing the disease is almost 100%. So, in this case, it might be important to know whether one carries the mutation or not. However, these cases are very rare.

What we see in the general population is sporadic Alzheimer's disease, which is much more common. The heritability of sporadic Alzheimer's disease is 75%, i.e., the contribution of the genome to the development of the disease is 75%. Please understand that this does **not** imply that a first degree relative will have a 75% probability of developing the disease. Heritability is a population-based value, and it cannot be used at an individual basis. There are several genes, and other non-genetic factors, which are related to the risk for developing sporadic Alzheimer's disease.

What do we know today? Not much more, but back in 1993 Alan Roses's group published a very nice paper [1]. In this study, they identified a variant of a gene called APOE. This gene has 3 alleles: it is present in 3 variants. Possession of the variant ε4, is related to an increased risk for Alzheimer's disease. What does this mean?

About 25% of a healthy control population carries the ε4 variant without suffering from Alzheimer's disease. However, in a group of AD patients almost 70% are APOEε4 carriers. Which means if you are a heterozygous carrier of ε4 variant, if you have one copy, or two copies (homozygous), you have a three-fold and eight-fold, respectively, increased risk of developing Alzheimer's disease. This finding has been broadly replicated and, therefore, it is considered stable.

However, if you look more closely at it – the sensitivity and specificity of this variant is only about 60%. This means there is absolutely no positive predictive validity when using this variant as a predictive factor. I remember when I was doing my residency in Bonn: there was this new lab sheet for clinical routine examination with a check box: 'APOEε4, yes or no?' I wondered why was that there? When I called up the lab the technician there told me it was for knowing whether the patient has Alzheimer's or not. However, this is absolutely the wrong implication of a ε4 genetic testing result. Indeed, the first Alzheimer's patient was not a ε4 carrier!

Remember, there might be a value in doing predictive genetics, but we need to understand how genetic information may be used and interpreted. Please keep also in mind, it is not only an issue of positive predictive values or sensitivity or specificity, there are other issues.

For instance, let us look at the interaction of the ε4 variant with the genetic background or ethnicity. If you are an ε4 carrier and you carry two copies and if you are of European ancestry: the odds ratio associated with this is 8, meaning you have about an 8-fold increased risk of developing the disease. If you are of sub-Saharan ancestry, you do not have any increased risk at all. If you are Japanese, and you are homozygous for ε4, you have a 33-fold increased risk of developing Alzheimer's disease. This means for a Japanese individual it might be important to know, and it is actually very informative to know, whether he/she is homozygous for ε4, whereas for a European it is less important, and for a sub-Saharan individual, it is absolutely irrelevant.

When talking about complex genetics, I truly cannot overstate the importance of the phenotype. Remember, complex human genetics is also a statistical discipline; one can correlate anything with anything. One could correlate genes with religious feelings, for example. In my opinion, the so-called God gene is absolutely meaningless. Scientifically speaking, it is simply correlating genetic variation with something, which we don't know what it is! This is not serious science.

Let us go back to understand why the choice of phenotype is important. I would like to stress that the value of genetics is realized only when it is combined with a suitable phenotype or trait.

What are the criteria for a suitable phenotype or trait? The trait should be heritable, be reliably assessable, and it should have a neuronal correlate (at least, in neuroscience) or a biological correlate. Human memory – the ability to remember episodes of our lives – is such a suitable biological trait. It is heritable, it can be reliably assessed and it does have a neuronal correlate.

Why do complex genetics on memory? Sometimes, we want to just know and understand the biology of this complex trait. If you want to understand in humans more about the biology of memory, not in model organisms, you can choose between two possible approaches. (1) The classical pharmacological approach: you think that a certain receptor or gene is important in memory, the first thing you have to do as a pharmacologist, you have to find a compound that will bind with the molecule that you are interested in, and then, to study humans to see whether they react and how they react when taking this drug, if their memory becomes better or not. This approach has its caveats (e.g. availability, safety, specificity). (2) The genetic approach: again, it might be hypothesis-driven for a certain receptor or gene related to human memory. Then, you scan in the human genome and look for genetic variants of this molecule. Some individuals would have a specific variant of the molecule, the other individuals have other variants, etc. You then can stratify it according to the groups with the different variants. If they significantly differ regarding the trait of interest (in this example, memory performance), then it is most probably due to the stratification that you did, i.e. it is due to the genotype. It is important to remember that these are group comparisons, not individual predictions.

If you study a group of students and measure their memory capacity, you will find a physiological phenotypic variability. Some students have good memory, and some do not. Importantly, studies in twins indicate that inherited factors account for about 50% of this variability. So, we know that this trait is heritable.

Imagine you are a student, and you are told to watch 30 words at a rate of 1 word per second, with the instruction to learn and recall them. In my presentation, I will now give an example of 10 words, and it is still quite challenging!

In any case, what you get is a normal distribution of performance. Some of the students remember nothing 5 minutes later; some remember 19 out of 30 words. This normal distribution is a good way to begin with a human genetics study. We conducted a hypothesis-based study first: we looked at the variants of the serotonin 2a receptor gene, either tyrosine or histidine. When we stratified the population we observed that tyrosine carriers had worse memory performance than histidine carriers.

Does this mean you have a bad memory if you are a tyrosine carrier? Absolutely not! However, what we learn from this study is that the serotonin 2a receptor is important for human memory function.

Thus, this genetic approach allows us to know and understand more about the biology, not about knowing one individual's fate. Today it is possible not to study just one variant but rather 900,000 variants of the genome in one individual. The standardized processing with genetic arrays and validated equipment really opens up a new era where we can study large populations. We now have the ability to scan the entire human genome and to identify variants, without a prior hypothesis, in order to understand more about biology and to not only look where the light is, but to look also where perhaps it is dark.

Can we use this strategy in Alzheimer's disease to identify molecules related to the pathological memory symptoms of this disease? In a genome-wide association study, we recruited 1,411 individuals and scanned their entire genome for 500,000 variants [2]. We identified a very high peak that was statistically significant; again, it was the ε4 variant of APOE that we saw before. In addition, it is important to understand that when you do 500,000 statistical tests as in this case, you have to correct for false-positive results. With this correction, one can be more certain that the association observed is not a spurious one.

Another group adopted a similar strategy with genetic information from 10,000 individuals; they identified two variants in two genes that were very highly significant, CLU and PECAN [3]. Does this mean that someone with these variants will develop Alzheimer's disease? Absolutely not! Remember, again, these are group comparisons not individual predictions. Let us look at the odds ratio related to these genes: 0.9, as reported in a similar study [4]. At an individual basis, these variants are not relevant for the risk of developing Alzheimer's disease. Why are they so significant in terms of the analysis done in this genome-wide association study? This is because of the large sample size of 10,000 individuals; however, as we learned previously, this doesn't mean that the risk (or odds ratio) might be high as well.

With this data and other confirmation studies, we now know that the CLU and PECAN variants are related to the pathways that may lead to Alzheimer's disease. Somehow, these variants interfere with the physiological metabolic pathway. Again, we learn more about biology – not about the individual risks –when analyzing genetic data in a population.

Perhaps we still don't know more about individual risk because we are analyzing our studies erroneously. The used methodology appears like this: we analyze each variant independently, one at time, and associate it with a trait od interest. This is simple, straight-forward, but often wrong. In reality there are so many genes and interactions in the genome, which are simply not accounted for, in the way we are currently doing the studies.

Whether complex genetics will be really useful also for individual predictions or not depends therefore on the development of new analytical methods and algorithms. It is still uncertain whether this will be ever possible – whether someday we will be able to predict who is going to develop what complex disease and when by just using genetic information. Personally, I think it is not possible, at least not with any meaningful accuracy at the individual level.

Another interesting approach is taking data from individuals and creating genetic maps, for example, all over Europe [5]. In this study, the authors scanned the genome as usual, with 900,000 variants per individual. In doing so, one can identify based on genetic information which is the ethnicity of the respective individual. This is simply a genetic map of ancestry, which absolutely corresponds to the geographical map of ancestry! We are able of course to identify many things with genetics, but to predict whether something is going to happen is scientifically a completely different story.

There must be other ways to perform our calculations. For example, what we have done in the past, we tried to identify clusters of genes related to certain diseases [6], instead of looking at only one variant at a time. In Alzheimer's disease we are, again, able to identify clusters of genes related to this disorder. But do they give us more information in terms of prediction? No, they don't: it looks better than one marker, but the sensitivity and specificity are still very low. So, still this cluster information is useful only for understanding biology, not for individual prediction.

In another study, we identified a cluster of genes related to 'good' human memory [7]. With this information, one can calculate an individual 'genetic score', which is how many of these genes or alleles are you possessing, weighted by their effect size. So, it's now possible to calculate your individual 'genetic score' for good memory! However, what does this really mean? It doesn't automatically mean that you have a good memory. We also observed that the higher the genetic score, the more activity in memory-related regions of the brain we can measure by functional magnetic resonance imaging (fMRI). However, this positive correlation is measurable only in groups. At an individual basis it is not relevant. We still have much to learn about the underlying biology.

We can use genetic information to understand the neural mechanisms of, for example, emotional memory. You often remember the more emotional events of your life than the neutral ones. One can test this ability and quantify a related phenotype by showing standardized photographs; most of the subjects are able to remember the more positive or negative pictures versus the neutral pictures. When we do this, we get a normal distribution of phenotypic variability and we can stratify the phenotype according to the genetic information. Therefore, we can learn about the biology of emotional memory.

We quantified this phenotype in 435 healthy Swiss participants and found a gene related to emotional memory, called the α2B-adrenergic receptor [8]. Carriers of a specific deletion variant of this gene have –as a group, not individually, better emotional memory than non-carriers.

We can do this analysis also for memories related to traumatic experiences, such as those leading to post-traumatic stress disease. To study this, we went to Rwanda and studied subjects who suffered from traumatic memories. These people were survivors of the genocide in 1993–1994 [8]. Again, the specific deletion variant of the α2B-adrenergic receptor gene was related to strong traumatic memories. This is a nice example of the real power of human genetics – you learn a lot about biology and sometimes also pathophysiology.

We can use the genetic approach to identify drug targets as well. It is a very valuable source of information. For example, we did a hypothesis-free scan of the entire genome to identify genes related to good human memory. We identified one gene, called KIBRA, which is related to memory performance; KIBRA is expressed in the human brain, and also it is related to differential brain activation on MRI [9].

When we looked more closely at KIBRA, we realized that KIBRA is related to a pathway called ROCK [10]. There are compounds that interfere with this pathway, such as hydroxyfasudil, and we know now that in aged rats, hydroxyfasudil improves memory. Today, hydroxyfasudil is being tested in phase I human clinical trials. This knowledge would not have come about without the ability to do hypothesis-free genetic studies simply because we didn't know about the existence of KIBRA before.

However, when talking about human genetics and the quest for 'personalized medicine', there are huge caveats with the current approaches and the results are prone to erroneous interpretations. Remember that the difference between group statistics and individual prediction is enormous. In addition, by exploring the human genome in this manner, we produce data sets that are huge. We receive new information from the Human Genome Project, which we use to help us understand more about biology, diseases, and health. Someday, this information will come to the healthcare society through education and/or training. However, it is still dangerous to leave it the way it is now: several other 'pillars' need to be considered before coming to an interpretation at the society level, such as ethics, legal, and safety issues. One has to avoid erroneous interpretations of human genetics, but the reality is, at the moment, these wrong interpretations are difficult to avoid.

Several companies offer services for 'personalized medicine', sometimes without any medical advice. The largest company right now is called 23andMe; on their website, you can either 'Fill in your family tree', 'Take charge of your health', or 'Choose to have it all'. If one focuses on 'Take charge of your health', the options are: 'Upgrade your health records with your carrier status', 'Live well at any age', or 'Get the treatment that's right for you'.

I went to the website myself after a colleague asked me whether I was in collaboration with this company (no, I am not). I wanted to know what he was talking about and focused on 'Upgrade your health records with your carrier status'. Then, I realized there is a complete list of traits and phenotypes, where supposedly you can know your genes related to this phenotype. They do not only include diseases but also, for example, measures of intelligence and memory. In other words, the company wants to help you know, whether you possess genes that are related to good memory.

At first, I thought who did this work on genes and human memory, I thought we did? The 23andMe website, in fact, says if you genotype this polymorphism and if you are carrier of the KIBRA T allele, then you have slightly increased episodic memory; they even cited our study! This is outrageous. First of all, you do not need a genetic analysis to know whether you have good episodic memory, you can test this yourself. Secondly, the interpration on this website is absolutely wrong! Thirdly, unfortunately, we can not do anything about this: it is published data, they just take this information and produce a test, with a false interpretation.

Another company called Psynomics tells you whether you have bipolar disease or not. This is wrong: as it was with memory, because bipolar disease is related many alleles, its of which with very little predictive validity. Then there is Neuromark, providing genetic markers of suicide ideation emerging from certain anti-depressants. All of these companies are based on mostly 'solid scientific data'; however, they have misinterpreted, or taken out of context, the meaning of these studies.

For example, Neuromark cites one well-conducted study that was published a couple of years ago and which clearly states in the abstract: "**If replicated**, these findings may shed light on the biological basis. . ." [of suicidality] ". . .and help identify patients at increased risk". If replicated. This is not the case, as this study has not been replicated. Still, this company claims that one can do this test to predict suicidality after the use of anti-depressants.

All of these companies address important issues, this is true, but the implications are not supported by the scientific data. There are some other issues. First of all, are the tests diagnostic or predictive? Is it a direct-to-consumer or direct-to-doctor test, who informs you about the implications? Mostly it is direct-to-consumer. This is dangerous – the consumers are a vulnerable population; furthermore, doctors often do not know what to do with this information, there is the possibility of a stigma for some of these disorders, and negative reactions can occur. There are many, many issues.

The so-called 'personalized medicine' offered by these companies only addresses one issue and does not explain everything; furthermore, it definitely should not be the case of a money-making scheme – like slick oil company executives – by taking advantage of consumers and oversimplifying what are truly complex issues.

We do need personalized medicine to understand biology and perhaps to help where ever we can. Eric Green, the Head of the National Human Genome Institute in the U.S., was recently asked about diagnosing the future of genomics, specifically, what advice would he have for people who are considering buying personal genomic services from a company to find out their genetic risk for common diseases? [11]:

"I haven't yet gone to get that information, because I think that the amount of information available at this time wouldn't really change anything that I am doing. A lot of what I know about my own health is based on family history – I think that understanding family history, and making sure your physician knows that, is incredibly valuable, and that's where I would put my priority at the moment. But, it is a changing landscape, so I don't think any advice I would give today would be the same a year from now."

I cannot agree more with Dr. Green's advice.

In my opinion, the real value of genetic research is using it as a tool to understand biology, everything else is secondary. So, what do you need 'personalized medicine' for? Do you need it for prediction? Might be, depending what you want to predict and depending on the consequences of this prediction. Do you need it for diagnosis?

Again, depending on what you want to diagnose and the implications. Do you need it for pharmacogenomics? Yes, for sure, but here, the implications are slightly different. It is a very different story to say: 'You have an 80% risk of developing breast cancer' versus 'You have an 80% risk of reacting bad to this medication'. As a doctor, if I know that the drug has an 80%-vs-20% efficacy, then this is okay, because the consequences – for the possibility of making a wrong choice – are often not as heavy with regards to a medication and its reactions (balancing risk and benefit), versus the consequences of having a wrong diagnosis or prediction, leading to wrong treatment and worse.

Questions and Answers

Q. [*Regine Kollek*]: We also have to consider the historical development in science itself. I don't know whether you remember, when the Human Genome Project started, the major players in the field really put forward all sorts of messages. Like – once we have analyzed the genome, we will be able to cure cancer, and to understand this and that. Then, we had the editorials from Nature and Science that we would even be able to solve the major social problems, and so on and so on. This was really put forward massively to the public and the politicians in order to get funding for the project. What we have to deal with right now is some sort of aftermath of this kind of message. What do you think?

A. [*Papassotiropoulos*]: I partially agree. In a sense, there was a kind of hype, as is always the case with human beings. If there is a new methodology that seems very efficacious, of course, there will be a hype. But not everything these colleagues said was wrong. The information from the HGP really helped to identify the drugs, which are absolutely efficacious. Think about some of the cancer drugs that are related to human genetic information, antibodies, and so forth. So there is a certain face value in claiming this. However, the hopes you might initiate when saying such can sometimes be quite disproportionate. This is our role – to dampen the optimism a bit or to show now what we think is the right way to go. Keeping in mind that this is a changing landscape, in a year from now I might be giving a completely different talk: that the real value of human genetics is prognosticating . . . whatever. I don't think that will be the case, but it is a changing landscape nevertheless.

Q. [*Manuel Battegay*]: Can you speculate a little bit about the delta, between the group results and the individual results? In the workshop this morning, we heard about epigenetics and activating and silencing genes. Will we be able to measure this on a large scale as well?

A. [*Papassotiropoulos*]: It really depends on the phenotype. I do think the addition of epigenetic information will be of tremendous importance in cancer, for some cancer phenotypes. There, you have the source or organ in your hands and you can really measure the tumor. It is a completely different story in neuroscience. Here, I don't think epigenetics will always help, at least in some neuroscience-related phenotypes, e.g. depression and anxiety. The tissue is difficult to get. But there are some neuroscience-related phenotypes where this epigenetic approach might work, so I would not be only pessimistic.

Q. [*René Spiegel*]: Some 10 days ago, we had Dr. Kurzweil talk here in Basel about futuristic things. He projects things into a few years, 10 years, and 20 years, to tell us what he thinks what will happen. He believes he will live a thousand years because he is taking all these measures to prolong his own life. Now Andreas, you tell us that it is absolutely impossible to get down to the individual level with genome-wide association studies. But what drives you in this research, I am sure, is the hope that we get down to the individual level. Isn't it just a matter of calculating power, to dissect this complexity of individuals, genes and interactions, to really get down to the individual level?

A. [*Papassotiropoulos*]: You are asking, in fact, what is the core of my message. What drives me is to know biology, to learn biology, this is number 1. Two, perhaps someday to identify mechanisms related to diseases of human cognition, and when it comes to the individual level, to prediction: As a scientist I don't think we will be able to get predictive values, sensitivity and specificity, beyond 80% in any neuropsychiatry-related complex phenotype, whatever we do with human genetics, even if we scan the entire genome. Then comes the question, what do you need this 80% for? So, we need to talk about the consequences of this 80%. I hope to reach individual levels of prediction when it comes, for example, to questions of response to a certain medication. But to predict who will have good memory 30 years from now is ridiculous. You cannot predict this at an individual level with sufficiant accuracy; you would need sensitivity and specificity levels well above 90% to be able to truly predict this kind of phenotype, which is influenced by nongenetic factors such as the environment. We are just unable for most phenotypes, whatever we do, to pass over a certain limit of sensitivity and specificity.

Q. [*Klaus Lindpaintner*]: Could you speculate: one of the overall themes of this conference is how will patients and their families deal with this prognostic information? We know from studies in Huntington's families that some individuals will do very well with it and some might not. This might influence the amount of information, or the 'right to know' or the 'right to NOT know'. Can you speculate if there might be some sort of phenotype, biochemical or genetic, that can say who is more likely to deal with the information better?

A. [*Papassotiropoulos*]: Absolutely, there is already a phenotype, which predicts how people respond to this. It has to do with whether you are Greek or Swiss! The way to deal with this information is different in Greece versus Switzerland. This is a prognostic marker at the group level. But honestly, for these kinds of very personal information, I don't think we will ever get down to the individual level. It is complex. This is the difference between group and individual.

References

1 Corder EH, Saunders AM, Strittmatter WJ, Schmechel DE, Gaskell PC, Small GW, Roses AD, Haines JL, Pericak-Vance MA: Gene dose of apolipoprotein E type 4 allele and the risk of Alzheimer's disease in late onset families. Science 1993;261:921–923.

2 Reiman EM, Webster JA, Myers AJ, Hardy J, Dunckley T, Zismann VL, Joshipura KD, Pearson JV, Hu-Lince D, Huentelman MJ, et al: GAB2 alleles modify Alzheimer's risk in APOE epsilon4 carriers. Neuron 2007;54:713–720.

3 Beecham GW, Martin ER, Li YJ, Slifer MA, Gilbert JR, Haines JL, Pericak-Vance MA: Genome-wide association study implicates a chromosome 12 risk locus for late-onset Alzheimer disease. Am J Hum Genet 2009;84:35–43.

4 Harold D, Abraham R, Hollingworth P, Sims R, Gerrish A, Hamshere ML, Pahwa JS, Moskvina V, Dowzell K, Williams A, et al: Genome-wide association study identifies variants at CLU and PICALM associated with Alzheimer's disease. Nat Genet 2009;41:1088–1093.

5 Novembre J, Johnson T, Bryc K, Kutalik Z, Boyko AR, Auton A, Indap A, King KS, Bergmann S, Nelson MR, Stephens M, Bustamante CD: Genes mirror geography within Europe. Nature 2008;456:98–101.

6 Papassotiropoulos A, Wollmer MA, Tsolaki M, Brunner F, Molyva D, Lütjohann D, Nitsch RM, Hock C: A cluster of cholesterol-related genes confers susceptibility for Alzheimer's disease. J Clin Psychiatry 2005;66:940–947.

7 de Quervain DJ, Papassotiropoulos A: Identification of a genetic cluster influencing memory performance and hippocampal activity in humans. Proc Natl Acad Sci USA 2006;103:4270–4274.

8 de Quervain DJ, Kolassa IT, Ertl V, Onyut PL, Neuner F, Elbert T, Papassotiropoulos A: A deletion variant of the alpha2b-adrenoceptor is related to emotional memory in Europeans and Africans. Nat Neurosci 2007;10:1137–1139.

9 Papassotiropoulos A, Stephan DA, Huentelman MJ, Hoerndli FJ, Craig DW, Pearson JV, Huynh KD, Brunner F, Corneveaux J, Osborne D, Wollmer MA, Aerni A, Coluccia D, Hänggi J, Mondadori CR, Buchmann A, Reiman EM, Caselli RJ, Henke K, de Quervain DJ: Common Kibra alleles are associated with human memory performance. Science 2006;314:475–478.

10 Huentelman MJ, Stephan DA, Talboom J, Corneveaux JJ, Reiman DM, Gerber JD, Barnes CA, Alexander GE, Reiman EM, Bimonte-Nelson HA: Peripheral delivery of a ROCK inhibitor improves learning and working memory. Behav Neurosci 2009;123:218–223.

11 Hayden EC: Diagnosing the future of genomics. Nature, November 23, 2009. DOI: 10.1038/news.2009.1102. http://www.nature.com/news/2009/091123/full/news.2009.1102.html

Prof. Dr. med. Andreas Papassotiropoulos
Division of Molecular Psychology
Life Sciences Training Facility, Biozentrum
University of Basel
Birmannsgasse 8
CH–4055 Basel (Switzerland)

Pfleiderer G, Battegay M, Lindpaintner K (eds): Knowing One's Medical Fate in Advance. Challenges for Diagnosis and Treatment, Philosophy, Ethics and Religion. Basel, Karger, 2012, pp 26–37

Ethical Decision-Making on Genetic Diagnosis Facing the Challenges of Knowing One's Medical Fate in Advance

Gabriela Brahier

UFSP Ethik, Ethik-Zentrum, Universität Zürich, Zürich, Switzerland

The possibilities of modern genetic diagnostics have led to major progress in the fields of disease diagnosis (diagnostic application) and disease therapy (therapeutic application). At the same time, the field of genetic diagnostics opens new possibilities for early detection of disease predispositions (predictive application); however, those affected have to face extensive decisional conflicts of a completely new manner. On the one hand, the so-called predictive genetic diagnosis promises more detailed and long-term information regarding the individual course of disease or health. On the other hand, patients are confronted, however, with the task of incorporating the importance of the predicted probability into their subjective outlook on life. The current possibilities opened up by predictive genetic diagnosis mean that the persons affected by it are facing new challenges with regard to their futures. Statistics relevant to one's state of health or disease need to be put into the context of one's own future plans. These people have to imagine a statistical probability as a potential way of living their own lives in a much stronger way, compared to people with a non-genetic medical prognosis.

This addresses an individual biographical aspect, in which medical ethics is becoming increasingly interested. Numerous studies investigate how affected individuals perceive genetic diagnostics and which psychological and emotional consequences the decision-making process involves (for example, see [1]). The importance of individual moral concepts is also repeatedly emphasized for the decision-making process (for example, see [2]). Since the 1970s, the principle of autonomous decision-making has established itself in order to help those affected to reach a decision (whether or not to use genetic diagnostics) conforming to their values. The patient should decide by himself/herself, if he/she wants to undergo genetic testing – and thereby risk a deeper insight into his/her own medical fate – or not.

However, comparably little notice is taken of the *value synthesis* strategy during decision-making. How do affected people deal with the possibilities of intensified future-related probability calculations and how do they come to decisions concerning genetic diagnostics conforming to their individual values? Or, in other words: what are distinctive characteristics of an autonomous decision? The answer to this question is equally relevant to those affected as well as to their consulting physicians.

The example of prenatal genetic diagnosis illustrates particularly well how the possibility of knowing one's medical fate in advance can influence individual decision-making processes; on the one hand, because pregnant women are often confronted with an unexpected risk diagnosis, which they have not yet been able to debate, and, on the other hand, because (due to the limited time of the pregnancy) decisions need to be made under particularly great pressure. Paradigmatically, the question that arises here is, how these women – whilst dealing with the predicted probabilities – come to a decision (concerning prenatal genetic diagnosis) that can be considered as their autonomous decision.

This question guides the following statements. Using the example of prenatal genetic diagnosis, I shall critically question and empirically examine the current principle of autonomous decision-making, before attempting a reformulation.

First of all, the model of an informed consent shall briefly be discussed in its function as a key to autonomous decision-making in the context of modern medicine. Secondly, an empirical study conducted by the author shall be presented. It analyzes ethical decision-making processes in women in conjunction with prenatal genetic testing and focuses their ways of dealing with the occurrence of knowing in advance. The results have major consequences for the theoretical concept of personal autonomy as well as for the practical model of nondirective genetic counseling, which will thirdly be discussed. These are supposed to be of high relevance for clinical ethics, if it is to be interested in the concrete values and decision-making processes of the concerned individuals.

The 'Informed Consent' Model as the Key to Autonomous Decision-Making

Potential horizons are always in the back of the mind of a pregnant woman making a decision with regard to prenatal genetic testing: *Will the child be handicapped? Would I be able to cope with a handicapped child? Should I go through with the genetic tests? What conclusions would I draw from the test results?*

Since the decision primarily affects the future plans of the woman concerned, as well as her family, medical counseling aims to facilitate a decision which harmonizes as closely as possible with her individual system of values. Achieving this is the purpose of so-called informed consent. On the basis of detailed information, together with nondirective counseling, the patient should be placed in a position where she can make an uninfluenced and self-determined decision. Comprehensive information about the test procedure, its risks and benefits should – or so the idea – facilitate and guarantee autonomous decision-making. Informed consent is recognized today as a binding standard in all areas of medicine (see [3]).

By all means, enabling those concerned to decide further medical steps by themselves should be viewed very positively. And yet, in recent times, various authors have called into question just how 'informed' such test decisions really are. Empirical studies from within the social sciences have shown that those involved in decision-making processes in conjunction with genetic testing often do not properly understand the information they receive and sometimes even consciously ignore it (for examples, see [4, 5]). These findings cast fundamental doubt on just how much information is taken in, or rather on the direct link between the imparting of comprehensive information and autonomous decision-making.

Now, one could say that women who pay less attention to imparted information are less autonomous in their decision-making. And yet, in the last few years even the principle of autonomy – developed chiefly and so enduringly by Tom Beauchamp and James Childress (see [6]) – has been subjected to intense criticism. This criticism states that an interpretation of autonomy based on the imparting of information assumes an isolated and rationalistically narrow concept, disregarding the social contexts of those affected, as well as the significance of their intuition for the decision-making process. Feminist ethics, in particular, has emphasized the role played by relationships and demanded that autonomy be reformulated as relational autonomy (for example, see [7]).

Such criticism gives rise to the conjecture that both the model of informed consent and its underlying principle of autonomy require reconsideration. Of course, the model of informed consent is primarily a legal model of a postulatory nature. During the debate, however, this fact is often buried in oblivion. For example, in Switzerland, the principle of self-determination in the context of genetic diagnosis has been enshrined in law in the 'Bundesgesetz über genetische Untersuchungen beim Menschen' (see [8]). This principle specifies a complete disclosure of all available information, as the basis for the patient for autonomous decision-making (as opposed to the paternalistic understanding in a physician-patient relationship). Thus, a decision is considered to be autonomous, if it has been made in full knowledge of the facts. However, this says little about the practicability of the principle. From a legal point of view, the acquisition of an informed consent model seems to be very valuable. But when put into practice, it hardly helps the patient deal with the received information in an appropriate manner. It cannot be legally required that those who are affected actually do include the received information into their own decision-making process.

In the following, the model of informed consent is not denied, but rather differentiated and supplemented in its reading. The thesis is put forward such that it has to be interpreted in a certain way, in order to be applied effectively and to also meet the normative requirements, empirically. That is why we primarily need to look at how autonomy needs to be perceived in order to do justice to the reality lived by those affected. How do these people deal with the received information? How do decision-making processes actually unfold, and when is a decision to be deemed autonomous? Let us take a look at this in practice.

Ethical Decision-Making Processes in Women in Conjunction with Prenatal Genetic Testing: an Empirical Study

During the first trimester of pregnancy (usually between the 11th and 14th week of pregnancy), the so-called first trimester screening takes place as a part of routine pre-natal care, as it is available in many different countries. During an ultrasound scan, the nuchal translucency of the fetus is measured. Additionally, the results of a blood test and the expectant mother's age are included in the child's risk calculation for chromosomal aberrations. A calculated risk of 1:300 or more means an increased risk for the child to be born handicapped. Afterwards, additional examinations (for instance, genetic tests) can be run, in order to obtain more information on the child's state of health.

The current possibilities of prenatal genetic diagnostics, in particular, amnio-centesis and chorion villus biopsy, offer helpful tools for the early detection of fetal abnormality (for example, Down's syndrome). On the other hand, how-ever, as a result of these 'additionally' provided screening programs, many preg-nant women find themselves facing decisions that are often of excessive demand. This can lead to psychological stress, which is not to be underestimated. Invasive diagnosis, for example, does promise better knowledge of the child's state of health. However, it cannot be carried out, without risk to the fetus. At the same time, dealing with the prognoses of prenatal diagnostics (that are ultimately based on probabilities) proves to be extremely complex for the women. What does it mean to have a probability of 1:280 of giving birth to a child affected by trisomy 21? In this case, the probability of having a handicapped child is certainly smaller than with a risk of 1:50. Then again, the figure is above the reference value of 1:300, which is considered an increased risk. The ultimate question is how these numbers can be incorporated into the personal life of those affected and how they interpret them.

It is almost impossible to solve the problem objectively. This means the women have to ponder in detail what they are ready to accept. For most women, the period of uncertainty between the genetic test and receiving its results is very distressing. Further steps of the decision are put off until after the results have been presented. Women therefore report that they maintained a certain distance to their pregnancy and to their unborn child until the test results were available. In this context, Barbara Katz Rothman created the term 'tentative pregnancy' (see [9]).

Future-orientated deliberations, such as what a handicapped child would mean for one's individual lifestyle, or if possibly an abortion could also be taken into account, are already existent before carrying out the genetic test. The insecurities with which a woman deals when facing her decision are therefore very intense, not only after, but especially before the genetic diagnosis. That is why the following study focused on women's ethical decision-making processes in regard to prenatal genetic diagnostics after a suspicious first-trimester screening. The results are presented after a few short methodological notes.

Between September 2008 and August 2009, I conducted a qualitative interview analysis of decision-making processes in conjunction with prenatal genetic testing. The study was supported by the Swiss National Science Foundation and arranged in collaboration with the University Hospital of Basel and the Cantonal Hospital of Bruderholz (Basel-Land), Switzerland. The conceptual design of the interviews was narrative. First, it focused on the entire spectrum of thoughts, images and feelings which play a role in the decision-making process. Second, women were specifically asked how they ultimately found their way through the thicket of different considerations and manifold influences to arrive at *their* decisions. The questioning was fundamentally norm-theoretical, examining the values of the women which guided their decisions. This aspect also constitutes the special profile of this study.

Overall, 6 interviews were evaluated in accordance with the grounded theory. They were recorded on tape and transcribed in anonymous form. Obviously, a database of 6 evaluated interviews is too small to draw generalized conclusions. Furthermore, it is characterized by high selectivity. The gathered data, however, can indicate how women deal with ethical decision-making conflicts in the specific situation of prenatal diagnosis and counseling. Thanks to this data, one can anticipate well-founded ideas as new approaches to the subject matter.

The data set at hand for the evaluation was as follows: of the 6 women, 3 had decided against genetic testing, 3 in favor of it – all of which involved a chorion villus biopsy. All 6 interviews were held very shortly after having decided about the test. At the time of the interview, all of the women were over 30 years old, 5 were older than 35, 3 were 40 or older.

It is not possible to present the results in full here, but I would like to give an insight, particularly into the way in which the women justified their decisions concerning genetic testing. I illustrate the points I wish to make using direct quotations from the interviews. All names have been changed.

It emerged that the considerations of the women, when deciding in favor of or against genetic testing, could be divided into 4 groups.

(1) First of all, the women thought about the various aspects of their ways of shaping their lives. Even before undergoing a test, they were already thinking about what it would mean for them personally to have a handicapped child. Would they still have enough time for their other children? Would they still have time for their partners?

What about their careers and time for themselves? With regard to a potential child with disabilities, the women also deliberated whether they would be able to find the strength and resources required to meet that child's needs.

Future-related questions such as what kind of possible impact a handicapped child would have on their own way of life show that the decision does not only affect an isolated, single area of life, in fact it affects all areas of life. This also indicates that an anticipation of individual lifestyle scenarios is highly relevant for the overall decision-making process. (This finding partly corresponds to a study by Irmgard Nippert, see [10]).

From an ethical point of view, the women asked themselves if they could be what they considered a 'good mother' for their children, respectively a 'good wife' for their partners, when having a handicapped child. Their individual perception of what a 'good mother' and 'good wife' is was mainly linked to the thoughts of being present for her child and partner and being able to protect the family.

Here is a quotation from a woman whom I have named Muriel. This is how Muriel perceived her duty as a mother in the decision-making process:

Muriel

"(. . .) Well, to think (. . .) what about . . . the child, that hasn't been born yet, but yet already exists. And if I . . . uh, have to focus on this second child, where does that leave my daughter, and can I still be a good mother for my daughter? (. . .) And, well, I also had the responsibility to ask myself, as to what extent I would be able to bear that, or do I have to make sure that this child, that's already here, well . . . that it's protected so to speak, well that was also very difficult for me. . ."

Therefore, at first, mainly value and preference conflicts seem to character-ize future-related thoughts (for instance, on the role as a mother) as Muriel's quote suggests.

(2) The second group consisted of considerations related to abortion. Here the women deliberated whether they would be able to go through with an abortion and whether ethical and moral standpoints would even 'allow' it.

Here are quotations from 2 women, whom I shall call Zoe and Caroline:

Zoe

"(. . .) I couldn't have lived with having had an abortion. (. . .) I probably would have suffered from depression. (. . .) I just knew I couldn't have a child aborted (. . .) I couldn't see myself as a judge, giving a 'thumbs up' or a 'thumbs down'."

Caroline

"(. . .) For me it's as if children who are like that [i.e. handicapped] for some reason (pause) would like to, or need to, have that experience, or whatever, and if I had an abortion I would be taking away that chance, that experience. . ."

What is interesting here is the type of argumentation used by Zoe and Caroline. Both arguments revolve around a particular image of themselves: Zoe does not wish to be seen as a judge. This would not tie in with her personality, would not fit. And Caroline, as a mother, believes it her job to give even a handicapped child the chance to be born. She does not wish to see herself as someone who has robbed a child of this chance. I shall return to this point in a moment.

(3) The third group comprised a collection of risk assessments, including deliberations about the risks involved in an invasive test, and the degree of disability one could theoretically cope with in a child.

As the results show, a decision for or against the test was essentially made based on considerations between a personal risk assessment on having a handicapped child and assessing the risks of the test. Some women were afraid that the invasive test might injure and thereby harm the unborn child.

Regarding the severity of the disability, the individual feasibility assessment was characterized by personal images and feelings as well as personal views on the quality of life. These thoughts were strongly connected to the deliberations in other categories.

(4) Finally, the fourth group contained various considerations regarding the importance of fellow human beings. Here, the interview participants deliberated what others might think of them, what level of support they might expect from their partners, and how much positive expectations they have in their doctors in the decision-making process.

Every woman questioned said that her partner was the most important person to figure in the decision-making process, and that she had also had intense exchanges with close friends or family. In contrast, her doctor was frequently perceived as a 'source of information' who did, however, have the power to encourage or discourage her significantly, depending on his/her manner and reaction.

Muriel, for example, said:

"(. . .) I had the impression that the (female) doctor was more nervous than I was. . ., I mean. . . she didn't know how to deal with the situation. . . and that made me feel nervous all over again."

All the aspects cited make it very clear that the thoughts, images, and feelings involved in the genetic testing decision are extremely varied and complex. Therefore, the question arises of how a decision is ultimately supposed to emerge from this bewilderment of deliberations: how exactly do women proceed in order to bring all their wishes, preferences and values together in one decision? Is there a strategy of synthesizing which is common to all women?

I think there is. I would like to use a case study to give a brief illustration of this point. Tanya is 40 years old, and, at the time of the interview, pregnant with her first child. She told us:

"(. . .) the niece of a friend of mine is a doctor and, when she was pregnant, she was so worried that she had everything tested. And then the child was born and it couldn't see or hear, and the brain didn't develop as it should, and the child is severely handicapped. It's not even clear whether or not all those tests might have caused it. You hear stories like that. I haven't met the woman myself, but. . .I'm more of a positive thinker myself."

A positive thinker – that is how Tanya sees herself. Unlike the other woman in her account, she herself does not need to undergo invasive testing because her decision is guided by the conviction that everything will turn out alright in the end.

Tanya's statement could, of course, be interpreted differently: precisely as a positive thinker she could undergo genetic testing and trust in the belief that her child would not be harmed by it. But for her, as she told us, the tests were 'too invasive'. This is how Tanya ultimately arrived at her decision:

"Maybe the fact of the matter is. . . maybe at the end of the day the decision you make is basically a gut feeling. So (. . .) it really was a gut feeling, (. . .) I know. I sometimes think about whether this decision was a gut feeling or not and then wonder, did I do the right thing? And then I think, yes, well maybe it wasn't the right thing, but it was the thing [the decision] that was most me."

'The decision that was most me' – in other words, the decision which suited her best – a motive which we also witnessed with Zoe and Caroline. The decision which most makes a woman feel that she is heeding all the various demands made of her: her partner, her other children, herself, her career, etc.

Muriel said something very similar:

"I believe that you can only understand why someone decides this way or that way if you understand the values which led to this decision (. . .) I felt that we had looked at the situation as a whole, and I liked that because, for me, the decision-making process depended not just on one or two points, but on everything which makes me what I am."

There really does seem to be a common synthesizing strategy. It is geared towards the idea of authenticity, i.e. a certain perception of oneself, of one's own values and one's individual ideas on how the future should look.

This conclusion seems obvious, and intuitively we are not particularly surprised by it. And yet, in the context of the autonomy debate its consequences are far-reaching. A decision regarding genetic testing was perceived by the women interviewed as their own, autonomous decision when it was 'authentic'. In order to assess how they could best heed the various demands made of them, the women played through in their heads various lifestyle scenarios. For example, they considered how they would live as families, how they would organize their professional lives and how they could fulfill their roles as mothers. It is this anticipative imagining of personal futures which underlies the decisions taken by these women regarding genetic testing. Their own, autonomous decisions appear to emerge step by step as they anticipate individual lifestyle scenarios.

What are the consequences of this conclusion for theory and practice?

Autonomous Decision-Making as a Liberal Slant on Shaping One's Own Future – Consequences for Theory and Practice

A practical conception of autonomous decision-making, as sketched above, proposes that an autonomous decision develops as a process. As the interview results suggest, this process involves anticipated ideas about potential individual lifestyles.

Instead of operating with a concept of autonomy prescribing that persons are fully informed and not influenced, it could be worth considering whether autonomous decision-making is not aimed precisely at opening up a potential for assessing oneself and one's own ideas about the future. Put another way: whether or not a decision could be deemed autonomous to the extent to which it is able to provide individuals with a potential for assessing themselves.

A view of autonomy and autonomous decision-making thus reformulated would impact the current counseling strategies. The current strategies assume that doctors act as neutral counselors in nondirective consultation. And yet, the interview study shows that doctors – purely as a result of their behavior and reactions – for example, to the results of a pregnancy scan, directly influence pregnant women in their decision-making process. This implies that doctors in counseling sessions definitely influence women patients in some way, whether this is their intention or not.

The broad range of role compulsions and personal self-projection in everyday life has already been described in the 1960s and 70s in the social sciences (primarily by the American sociologist Erving Goffman, see [11]). Ever since this, in German-speaking areas, sociologists – such as Ulrich Beck or the social psychologist Heiner Keupp (for example, see [12]) – have been examining the complex issues of everyday life. They have impressively demonstrated that an autonomous self-sufficient lifestyle, unaffected by outside influences, does not comply with the practical life-world anyway.

If this observation is wholly or partially correct, a shift in the conception of genetic counseling can also ensue (see [13, 14]). It is then no longer paramount that women receive comprehensive information in order to make uninfluenced decisions. Far more, it is paramount that a woman can view a decision as her own decision, one which pays best possible heed to all the aspects which are relevant for her. Thus, understanding information no longer only means correctly comprehending the information itself, but being able to apply it to the context of one's own life.

This viewpoint would give doctors the liberty to provide proper counseling. Counselors would no longer need to restrict themselves to imparting information, but could openly help patients to reach their own, autonomous decisions in harmony with their own values. It could be a large benefit for every individual concerned if the counselor's role is going to change from the one of a pure informant to that of a real companion.

The next question arises of how to help a woman to reach such a decision. On the basis of the interview study, my proposal would be: by helping her to play through various lifestyle options in her head, imagine future scenarios anticipatively, and sketch out her own life story.

Would genetic counseling, comprehended in this way, still be a job for doctors? Or would we need to consider developing a new profession for this field? What role could be played by psychologists or hospital chaplains? This area provides great potential for further research. The future mission of medical ethics just might be to emphasize individual decision-making processes, not to let them turn into radical individualism, but rather, to speak openly on the question of values and constantly consider personal material traditions.

Questions and Answers

Q. [*Georg Pfleiderer*]: Regarding this reflection on 'my own identity' or 'my own authenticity': at what stage of the decision-making process did that occur according to your study? In one of the cases you were referring to I got the impression that it was rather a *reflection* that came *after* the process of the real decision making as a kind of summarizing me to self-reflection.

A. [*Brahier*]: During interviews, I had the impression the women did this [actively] – they were thinking about it all the time. Maybe in the interviews, it was more obvious because they had to think about and talk about it. In the end, as they said, they made it anyway. This is how they would have reached their decision, even if they had not talked to any doctor or to me for the study. They talk to their friends, their husbands – these aspects are very important to them.

Q. [*Klaus Lindpaintner*]: Do you think it would make a difference if the information content of the testing was different? In other words, obviously, all these prenatal tests have a certain degree of precision. Now, if those tests were a lot more precise and a lot more predictive do you think the responses would be different?

A. [*Brahier*]: This is a really interesting point. In my sample, there were women who were without any danger – really; they were in no serious danger of having a handicapped child. So, they had a chance of 1 in 3,000 or something like that, and they decided not to go for the invasive test. Anyway, they had the same model of going through all these various aspects and thinking about how they would like to lead their individual life. This was interesting in this very few sets - 6 interviews. The process was the same in the women with severe risk and with those with no risk at all.

Q. [*Peter Sebastian*]: Is there any data that compares the decision-making process between the paternal and maternal side? Is there a phase of individual counseling then joint counseling? How does that work?

A. [*Brahier*]: I can't speak from the counselor's perspective. I think this depends on the doctors, if they have talks with both parents. I decided to have the interviews with just the women, as I think it would have complicated the whole setting if I would have asked the men as well. I don't oversee the whole field, but I know of more empirical research with women and their concerns than those of the husband.

Q. [*Isabelle Filges*]: More a comment than a question: you asked would it be more appropriate for psychologists or medical ethicists to conduct these counselings because they are better equipped to integrate the autonomy and the life vision of the woman. Actually, the question then becomes, would they be able to transfer the medical information correctly, in all terms? I think it very much depends on the doctor who does the counseling, because this approach is already integrated into the genetic counseling that we do in our discipline. So, I think it is a matter of training of the doctors or the person who counsels. In other countries, like Great Britain or the United States, there are specifically trained genetic counselors from different backgrounds, especially for this field. I think it is not a matter where you come from, but that you have both the ability to foresee this integrated approach and to see all the details of the specific medical information it is necessary to deliver.

A. [*Brahier*]: Thank you very much, yes. The women told me that some doctors already carry out this type of discussion with patients and they say they feel it is really good. But not all, so it is very individualistic. I think it could be a good thing if doctors could be released from this pressure – that they **must** only give information and not advice – some do it anyway but others do not. Whether this could be of help is just on a very theoretical basis.

Another very important point: I didn't see it as an alternative. I think it doesn't in any way or any sense put medical or genetic counseling into question. Rather, it could be an additional offer that could help women reach decisions that are really their own.

[*Final comment: Filges*] In my experience, patients often ask to compare the risks. You talked mainly about the first-trimester screening risk, and when they have a high risk, like 1 in 280 as you mentioned, they ask to compare this risk to the risk of abortion due to an invasive procedure which is also 1 in 200, basically the same. Then you can have the discussion that one cannot compare the two risks, it is not simply numbers, a mathematical comparison, one has to really consider each decision personally, in terms of the consequences in their personal life as well as for their future life.

References

1   Marteau T, Richards M (eds): The Troubled Helix: Social and Psychological Implications of the New Human Genetics. Cambridge, Cambridge University Press, 1996.
2   García E, Timmermans DR, van Leeuwen E: The impact of ethical beliefs on decisions about prenatal screening tests. Searching for justification. Soc Sci Med 2008;66:753–764.
3   Faden RR, Beauchamp TL: A History and Theory of Informed Consent. New York, Oxford University Press, 1986.
4   Michie S, Dormandy E, Marteau TM: Informed choice: understanding knowledge in the context of screening uptake. Patient Educ Couns 2003;50:247–253.
5   Scully JL: Time, tests, and moral space; in Pfleiderer G, Rehmann-Sutter C (eds): Zeithorizonte des Ethischen. Zur Bedeutung der Temporalität in der Fundamental- und Bioethik. Stuttgart, W. Kohlhammer, 2006, pp 151–164.
6   Beauchamp TL, Childress JF: Principles of Biomedical Ethics. New York, Oxford University Press, 2001.
7   Mackenzie C, Stoljar N (eds): Relational Autonomy. Feminist Perspectives on Autonomy, Agency, and the Social Self. New York, Oxford University Press, 2000.
8   GUMG, in force since 01 April, 2007.
9   Rothman BK: The Tentative Pregnancy. Prenatal Diagnosis and the Future of Motherhood. New York, Viking Press, 1986.
10 Nippert I: Psychosoziale Folgen der Pränataldiagnostik am Beispiel der Amniozentese und Chorionzottenbiopsie; in Petermann F, Wiedebusch S, Quante M (eds): Perspektiven der Humangenetik: medizinische, psychologische und ethische Aspekte (in German). Paderborn, Ferdinand Schöningh, 1997, pp 107–126.
11 Goffman E: The Presentation of Self in Everyday Life. New York, Doubleday, 1959.
12 Keupp H, Ahbe T, Gmür W, et al: Identitätskonstruktionen. Das Patchwork der Identitäten in der Spätmoderne (in German). Reinbek bei Hamburg, Rowohlt, 1999.
13 Elwyn G, Gray J, Clarke A: Shared decision making and non-directiveness in genetic counselling. J Med Genet 2000;37:135–138.
14 Manson NC, O'Neill O: Rethinking Informed Consent in Bioethics. Cambridge, Cambridge University Press, 2007.

Dr. Gabriela Brahier
UFSP Ethik
Ethik Zentrum
Universität Zürich
Zollikerstrasse 117
CH–8008 Zürich (Switzerland)
Tel. +41 44 634 85 13, E-Mail brahier@ethik.uzh.ch

Ethical and Juridical Perspectives

Pfleiderer G, Battegay M, Lindpaintner K (eds): Knowing One's Medical Fate in Advance. Challenges for Diagnosis and Treatment, Philosophy, Ethics and Religion. Basel, Karger, 2012, pp 38–49

Mastering Familial Genetic Knowledge: Shared or Secret? Issues of Decision-Making in Predictive Genetic Testing

Anne Brüninghaus[a] · Rouven Porz[b,1]

[a]Research Center for Biotechnology, Society and the Environment (BIOGUM), University of Hamburg, Hamburg, Germany and [b]Ethics Unit in the University Hospital in Bern, Switzerland

Due to its predictive and statistical nature, genetic knowledge is often regarded as a 'special' kind of knowledge. In this chapter, we emphasize the 'special' quality of genetic knowledge that does not only concern the individual, but the family as a *whole*. Thus, we reflect upon inner-familial conflicts, as the expectations towards and practices of dealing with knowledge and non-knowledge might diverge within a single family.

In general, the notion of 'genetic tests' refers to *all* procedures of molecular biological analysis that result in various statements about the heritable constitution of organisms [1, 2]. Genetic tests can be used to confirm a medical diagnosis if the patient already suffers and shows symptoms. Another prominent application is prenatal diagnosis, examining the genetic constitution of the foetus during pregnancy, or even preimplantation diagnosis, in the field of reproductive medicine. Predictive testing focuses upon the probability of whether a patient will develop a disease in the future (or not); it aims to detect dispositions for potential diseases. For example, a daughter whose father died of the neurological condition Huntington's disease can undergo predictive testing to ascertain her own disposition and obtain knowledge about her individual risk of getting the deadly disease.

Huntington Again

The reader might think: Huntington again? Yes! Huntington has been used as one of the most prominent examples to illustrate the ethical, social and legal implications of

---

[1]   Authors are listed in alphabetical order.

testing possibilities since the late 1990s (some benchmarking works include [3–5]). There is still no treatment for Huntington's, thus a decision in favour of predictive diagnosis cannot be justified simply for therapeutic reasons. Furthermore, predictive testing possibilities for Huntington's disease cannot easily be framed within the general arguments of medical decision-making. However, when the testing was made available in 1993, it was assumed that family members at stake might wish to find out about their disposition and might want to make use of the new genetic knowledge that is offered by the testing possibility (for example, see [6]). As prominently shown in the literature, people of affected families did not take up the test as often as anticipated by the scientists in the early 1990s. Family members developed sophisticated ways to deal with the potential knowledge of the disease and investigations of decision-making processes for or against taking a predictive test showed great flexibility in individuals' meaning-making (for example, see [7]).

In this article, we aim to examine the patterns behind the coping strategies for knowledge and non-knowledge, combine this insight with an analysis of how individuals deal with the arising inner-familial conflicts, and take a look at the existential dimensions of Huntington's (compare [8]): the 'outbreak' of the disease slowly but radically and inevitably changes the person concerned. Once the test result is found positive, with a penetrance of 99%, the certainty of developing the disease without prospect of a treatment or cure weighs down upon the affected person. One can hardly imagine a more 'existential' case of a disease. So how do people cope with the possibility of the predictive test? From a philosophical point of view, do they want to 'know'? Do they want to find 'certainty' in the conduction of the test? Or do they actively decide against this seemingly uncertain knowledge of a certain predictive test? And how is their whole biography influenced by this necessity to decide?

In order to be able to account for both the internal argument and the ethical aspect of dealing with knowledge and non-knowledge in decision-making, we deploy a twofold methodological approach to analyse an interview transcript of a testing decision of a female interviewee whose father had died of Huntington's.

We start by giving some methodological insights to our approach, then, we summarise the interview story for the reader. The first analysis by Anne Brüninghaus reconstructs patterns of the individual's biography that lie behind the different strategies of dealing with knowledge about the disease in the family. Then, Rouven Porz uses an interpretative approach to philosophically question some core features in the process of decision-making from a normative ethical point of view. Both authors conclude and summarize the findings in an interdisciplinary conclusion.

Methodological Approach

The interview with 'Mrs Alberta' is part of the first author's PhD project on decision-making for or against a genetic test of people at risk for hereditary diseases. The verbal data was captured using narrative interviews [9]: each interviewee was prompted to tell his or her 'story' of the decision from their own perspective. Pseudonyms are used in the transcription for all names, places and locations, and the reported dates are altered. The main part of these interviews was narrated without interruption by the interviewer ('main story'). The second part of the interview ('inquiry part') consists of questions by the interviewer that aim to clarify or extend on parts of the main part, and of a number of theory-based general questions.

Two different methodologies are combined here in order to create an interdisciplinary perspective of analyzing decision-making processes. The first part of the analysis focuses on reconstructing of how the interviewee uses biographical events in creating a consistent representation of the past and how these events then become part of an individual's biography. Basis for this approach is the idea of narrative-analytical interpretation, a biographical research method developed by Fritz Schütze [10]. The order of biographical events is analyzed to identify individual patterns or principles of dealing with different situations. The interviewee's individual narrative structure also exposes patterns that progress over time to enable him or her to deal with ongoing new and unknown situations. The second part of the analysis uses an interpretative phenomenological approach (IPA) [11]. The aim of IPA is to understand in-depth the perspective for individuals affected, starting from the interview text. The interpretative analysis is then linked to a normative ethical argumentation.

Of course, both methodological approaches have similar background assumptions, focusing, for example, on the narrative of the interviewee or admitting that the researcher might come up with different interpretations than the interviewee him- or herself. Still, our two-fold analysis can show that the different perspectives on interpretations enrich the findings of an interview story.

The Story of Mrs Alberta – Our Overview[2]

Mrs Alberta is a married mother of two children in her forties. Within her family, she is the first one who decided to undergo predictive genetic testing for a disposition to Chorea Huntington. Her decision appears to have been a quite spontaneous one: Mrs Alberta herself calls it a 'kamikaze action' (for an overview of different patterns of learning about Huntington's disease in the family, see [12]). At a time when her brother started to develop potential symptoms of the disease, the diagnosis of Huntington's suddenly became a very concrete possibility for her own future.

[2] Building on narrative and interpretative methods we ask the reader to bear in mind that we can only provide here 'our story' of 'Mrs Albertas story'. We depict and combine certain elements from the interview to introduce her story in a coherent way. However, she herself might have done that differently.

Longing for knowledge, she quickly decided to have a predictive test. As her result was negative, Mrs Alberta was very relieved to not have entailed the autosomal-dominant disease on her children. Her brother was genetically tested a short time later and, in contrast to Mrs Alberta, tested with a positive result: his test confirmed the symptoms as part of Huntington's disease. (This lies within the complexity of genetic information that even a negative test result has lasting impacts on the family [13]).

There are also other incidences of Huntington's in the extended family. Mrs Alberta's cousin, her father and her aunt (her father's twin sister) had died of Huntington's disease about 20 years ago. But no one in the family ever spoke about the possibility of a hereditary disease nor even mentioned the term 'Chorea Huntington'. However, after having received the result of her own gene test, she unexpectedly learned that her mother had known about Huntington's already for a long time – since the very moment her father had gotten ill. Yet, the knowledge of the disease was being kept secret from the whole family – up to the very day of Mrs Alberta's brother's developed symptoms. Practices of dealing with genetic knowledge are known to differ widely between families, see [14].

The interview primarily covers her family history, the decision to undergo the test, her activities in a self-help group and her own private thoughts on Huntington's disease that formed from coping with her family's fate. She often emphasizes her attempt to openly deal with the familial disease.

Biographical Approach: 'Revelation' by Familial Genetic Knowledge and Dissociation from the Parental Generation

The contrast between knowledge and non-knowledge about her genetic disposition plays an elementary role in Mrs Alberta's narrative. This dichotomy is exemplified by two oppositional ways of dealing with Huntington's as a hereditary disease: that of the parental generation in the past, and that of Mrs Alberta in the present. The former is marked by non-communication within the family as a central pattern of action. This is referred to by Mrs Alberta as 'under the pledge of secrecy' (original language, *Mäntelchen der Verschwiegenheit*). As she structures her experiences, Mrs Alberta contrasts this motive over and over again with her own interaction with the disease: "it was for me in this moment really clear, perfectly clear, that I will do that [the genetic test, AB], and that *I want to know*, it was like that".

Mrs Alberta begins her impromptu biographical narrative with a sequence where she talks about the first symptoms of her aunt as her first point of contact with Huntington's. Rather rapidly, she recounts the second encounter with Huntington's: "and the second was always so, why does nobody say something about that. Because, that was somehow like that in the family, it's probably like that for many, everything somehow under the pledge, eh. Pledge of secrecy."

In this sequence, Mrs Alberta articulates that in the past, it was common practice in the family to keep things secret and prevent the disease from becoming a subject of discussion. Asking for a rationale for this behaviour, she demonstrates at the same time her understanding for the speechlessness in the family. At this point, feelings of being surrendered to the behaviour in the family surface for the first time, a behaviour that she could not change: "and *no one ever* said *something*, only *at some point* the term rheumatic joints was dropped". While her father's and aunt's disease was "so a really hefty period" for Mrs Alberta, she herself seems to have noticed the disease only in passing: "and, em, I in principle took that on only in passing [. . .] I don't know, why I never asked. Or I was too much involved with my own affairs, I don't know". On the one hand, Mrs Alberta is incapable of remembering all the events that took place in the family. On the other hand, she clearly remembers that she felt strongly affected. Thus, it is clear that during this time, Mrs Alberta kept to herself very much, and either could not or did not want to deal with the familial disease. She seems to have felt to have little influence on her family's life in the past, but it becomes clear that at the time of telling her story, her perspective has changed.

Mrs Alberta was obviously strongly affected by the experience of her father's disease. A moment of being overwhelmed is apparent when she herself feels a desire to have children: as she combines the experience of her father's disease with her own wish for having children, she develops a notion that the disease is of hereditary nature, realizes the possibility of a personal affectedness, and the possibility of having passed this disease to her unborn child: "Then, my father died [year], and, em, I have yes, during that time I have considered [. . .] becoming pregnant somehow, and then I went that far, and then I had, yes, such this miscarriage in the eighth week and then I have especially again// [truncated] this seemed somehow to surface again." Thereupon, Mrs Alberta questioned her mother again, who answered "that was assumed to be a hereditary disease eh, but it was impossible to verify. [I: Hm] What was true, because the gene test wasn't available at that time, eh."

At a point in time that is important to her, Mrs Alberta restates her doubts about the disease to her mother again and hopes for more clarity – especially since the miscarriage she had been starting to think about it. In this situation, her mother's statement seems to have put her to rest, and allowed her to realize her wish to bear a child: "which then relieved me, which was when I started the project kids".

In the following sequence, the topic of uncertainty surfaces as Mrs Alberta compares the behaviour of her brother with that of her father: "and as then was no more, then I really cried, and I said, somehow my brother reminds me so of my father, somehow, I have the feeling there is something". Here, the feeling of being overwhelmed that she suffered during her father's and her aunt's disease surfaces again. And again, she let herself be put to rest, this time by her husband.

But then, a friend of her brother's advised and made sure that he visited a neurological doctor. And it is this doctor who confirms what Mrs Alberta had repeatedly been suspecting before letting herself being calmed down: after a symptomatic diagnosis, the doctor speaks to Mrs Alberta's mother who suddenly confirms: "yes, my husband had Huntington's". Her mother further reports that she knows that it was Huntington's since her husband fell ill, and rationalizes her secrecy by stating that Mrs Alberta otherwise would not have had children. For Mrs Alberta, this starts everything all over again: her anxieties, her doubts – and her wish to acquire certainty by knowledge. With this desire for clarity she becomes, however, deeply disappointed as she experiences her mother's statement as avoiding the issue. Her mother's keeping secret of her father's diagnosis now adds on to holding back the symptoms of her aunt and her father. At this point, she desires clarity, openness and transparency, and wishes to develop patterns for dealing with the disease that stand in obvious contrast to those of her parental generation.

Trying to cope with her mother's behaviour, Mrs Alberta begins to develop arguments for carrying out a genetic test: "it was a very brief time, until I came to this gene test from this revelation until there, and I thought if I don't learn that now for me, then, eh, I start thinking myself ill". With these arguments, Mrs Alberta dissociates herself openly from her mother's behaviour; from the practice of secrecy, she shifts to taking action and goes as far to name her mother's statement a 'revelation'. While this can simply refer to the light thrown on the nature of the disease, an element of the stupefying unexpected is also present: there is exposure, but there is also hope. Therefore, this part of the narration is a central place of both being overwhelmed and of change: from the shock of the revelation to the reawakened spirit for action. This is a relevant argument of Mrs Alberta, for her own development as well as for her decision-making process.

Her wish for immediate certainty makes Mrs Alberta use the term Kamikaze to describe her path of action: "somehow I have [. . .] then decided for that and have let it made immediately. [I: Hm.] But that was rather a Kamikaze action, basically". Here, Mrs Alberta makes a point that while she took to genetic counselling, she always focused on the aspect of wanting to know. Only as an afterthought she realizes that her quick decision for a genetic test also bears negative consequences for her – consequences that she was in principle aware of but had shielded from herself in the decision process.

The process of making the decision for the genetic tests does not appear to take place only during the time when she was confronted with its immediate possibility. Instead, the intrinsic changes of perception and self-perception (e.g. initiated by her mother's 'revelation') had been taking place in her past. Her narration suggests that these changes formed a basis on which the quick and possibly intuitive decision for the test was made. These changes enabled Mrs Alberta to bring herself to say "I want to deal with that" and "come on, eh, take your life back, it goes on".

Mrs Alberta contrasts her own way of dealing with the disease with that of her family: over and over, she distances herself from the behaviour of her 'parental generation'.

By remembering her own change towards the behaviour of her family, she provides structure to her present story through patterns of the past. She thus uses this past in her current situation to deal with this delicate and painful situation and thus to make the choice for or against the genetic test.

Interpretative Phenomenological Approach (IPA) and Emerging Bioethical Issues

Methodologically speaking, we now continue with the interpretation, but we focus on the point of view of the second author. Interestingly, in spite of another method used, there will be some repetitions and relations to the first part of the interpretation. However, the following interpretation primarily aims to use Mrs Alberta's case as a potential illustration of the moral dilemma within families. From an ethical perspective, a detailed analysis of just *a single* case can heuristically help to evaluate and rethink potential ethical problems and consequences. These potential problems can then be discussed in and related to more general normative issues.

Restarting with the test decision, and as already shown above, Mrs Alberta quickly decided to undergo a predictive test as soon as she became aware of the potential disease of her brother. However, her brother's unstable health condition was not totally new to her. She explained this in the interview:

"[My brother] had become quite slow, and – ehm – he often did not manage to finish his work, and – eh – in addition, there were some rumours, he might be an alcoholic. (. . .) he is a bit, a bit weird somehow – ehm – speaking of his psyches, you know (. . .)."

In the course of her brother's first medical encounters, his doctor had also talked to their mother, and the mother obviously confirmed that her husband has suffered from similar symptoms. And actually, the mother seemed to know more about the father's disease than her daughter – Mrs Alberta – was aware of. This was more than surprising or rather shocking for Mrs Alberta as her mother had never openly spoken about the father's disease or death. Mrs Alberta says about the hidden knowledge of her mother:

"(..) I don't know, somehow, maybe, that is the way the generation [of my mother] acts, or maybe it is just a peculiarity of my mother (. . .) somehow we never ever talked about it."

Her mother had obviously worried that her daughter Mrs Alberta would decide against having children, would be afraid of the family disease, and she wanted to prevent her daughter from not having children. So the mother decided to keep silent about the family story.

"My mother said: I would not have grandchildren now, if I had told you before."

One might find this conscious silence as ethically disturbing: is a mother supposed to act like this? Or was she responsible for disclosing any details of the potential disease to her daughter? And if she was responsible to disclose, when was a good time to do so? Of course, possible answers to these questions would morally judge the mother's actions and we do not aim at doing this here. But what we can do is looking at the story even more closely. The mother said "then I would not have grandchildren now", so she had apparently tried to anticipate her actions. She probably kept thinking: what if I keep silent? What if I tell them? Disclosing the truth might have lead to a different reproductive life of her daughter, and perhaps, she just wanted to anticipate her daughter with children of her own. This anticipation made her become silent about the disease. However, this is not a lonesome decision – it is an act of consequence, and it affects the whole family structure. In addition, this conscious silence can only hardly be framed in terms of genetic counselling. Genetic counselling – at least from a bioethical perspective – often talks about confidentiality, autonomy or data protection. But in our case, it rather illustrates the difficult nets of kinship, it rather sheds light on issues of guilt and/ or loyalty toward family members, and it shows the limits of private identities and decision making [15]. Clearly, in our case at hand, one might argue that Mrs Alberta would have expected more loyalty from her mother. She might have expected to know more about her father. She at least wants to act loyal towards her own daughters:

"(. . .) so I quickly had the test done (. . .) there are my own children, and I kept thinking, I need to know, I need to know for my children, and – of course – I also need to know for myself (. . .)".

She does not use the notion of 'loyalty' here, but she asks for a new kind of transparency. The familial net of inherited disease needs to be tackled in transparency, not in discreet or obscure silence. So we can interpret her step towards the genetic test as a first step of clarity, a way to oneness and transparency:

"Bloody hell, I was so afraid to go for the test, but then I thought, no,– ehm – you deal with this now, (. . .) and you will deal with it openly (. . .)."

From the viewpoint of social anthropology, Monica Konrad describes similar issues of guilt and responsibility in Huntington families in her book *Narrating the New Predictive Genetics* [16]. She speaks of "home truths" (59ff) of each family and she explains the complexity of loyalty by stating that we cannot do justice to the complexity of the genetic counselling situation if the individual family member is considered separately from his or her relations. So, new forms of kinship dependencies do arise.

So, what was the mother supposed to do? There might be also good moral reasons to keep silence about the father's disease. Christoph Rehmann-Sutter [17] introduces the term of 'Zukunftsvergessenheit?' to the debate (a conscious forgetting/suppressing of the coming future). He talks about parents who should help their children to keep innocent about their own future. Of course, these questions can hardly be tackled in general ways, each family and context might be different, each 'home truth' comes with different webs of responsibilities [16]. But Mrs Alberta wants to rewrite her own 'home truth'. She wants to get rid of her parent's old home truth and create a new one – a more open one – in her own family. She wants openness and transparency in the way they deal with the potential disease. That is working for them, as her own children are encouraged to talk about the symptoms of the mother's brother quite openly.

"(. . .) the kids were still very young, but one day, one of them came up to me and said: Mom – can you make a jump? And I was thinking, what? Yes, please jump. And then I hopped and she said: Okay. You can do that, but your brother he can't. I asked him, but he could not jump."

Of course, these are children's words, but they illustrate a new openness in their home truth: the brother of her mother is not able to 'make jumps' anymore. Somehow, he is suffering from a disease that keeps him from acts such as jumping around with the kids. Quite clearly, Mrs Alberta wants her kids to know the 'truth', as she herself was missing truth for too long: "Being lied to, and nobody had told me the truth, so my mother could not tell me the truth? And I kept thinking, I just want to know the truth."

For her, the possibility of the genetic test was a chance for truth: "So I went to this geneticist (. . .) and I did the test immediately."

From a bioethical perspective, it is interesting to think about the perception of a genetic test. For Mrs Alberta, the test was a way to the truth, the kind of truth that her own mother was not able provide to her. And, to state the very obvious: the *patient* Alberta must have been convinced that she can *rely* on the test. She must have believed in genetics, she thought that she can find 'truth' in her genes. In his latest book, Hub Zwart talks about *De waarheid op de wand* (the 'truth on the wall') [18]. He provocatively alludes to the rise of medical technologies of imaging. Nowadays, the diagnostic 'truth' about the patient is found in imaging; the modern (or postmodern) doctor does not need to look at the patient anymore, he can analyse the medical image of the patient on the wall or computer screen. The visible and embodied patient shifts to the background in the decision-making processes. We can make the same analogy to the field of molecular genetics. Medical 'truth' is now inherited, it can be found in our genes. Of course, patients must be able to relate to this abstract knowledge; they must be able to make sense of it. Mrs Alberta clearly did.

Still, one might find it reassuring to see that in our case such 'home truth' stories can make sense without genetic knowledge. The kids of Mrs Alberta were too young to make sense of the genetic disposition of the ill brother. Still, they could make sense of his symptoms. From their perspective, it was maybe the man who could not jump while they were playing. This is not as trivial as it may sound at first sight. It just shows that we need a variety of explanations to come to the same 'truth'. In parallel to medical 'truths' we need to have coherent and consistent 'truths' in our home lives. We need to make sense of testing. A negative result of a predictive test stays invisible in our home life. You cannot really grasp it, you cannot make it visible for your children (of course, you can explain it, but the children will not have a lively picture of it, they will not have personal experience with it). From a normative ethical point of view, the different ways of finding 'truths' should be balanced carefully. What for one person might count as truth might be ungraspable for the next. What for one family constitutes truth might be unloyal behaviour for the next one. This clearly challenges genetic counselling, but at the same time, it makes genetic knowledge relative. We need to create meaning first – genetic knowledge can help, but we can also come to meaningful solutions without genetic knowledge.

Conclusion

Our case study clearly suggests that decision-making in the context of genetic diagnostics cannot be understood as an individual process concerning only a single person at-risk – the consequences of a decision involve the *family as a whole*. This is also true for the interaction with genetic knowledge – this knowledge is not 'owned' by a single individual, it is shared between *family members*.

Methodologically speaking, we made a case for interdisciplinary work and combined different interpretative perspectives [19], concretely: the results of biographical narrative analysis and IPA. These two perspectives clearly complement each other as they both share a focus on the individual and thus increase the validity of the findings: values of knowledge shared or not shared in a family.

Huntington's disease is a textbook example in the discussion of predictive testing. However, at the moment public health genomics and the focus on polygenetic diseases do raise new questions, for example, regarding the need to alter patients' lifestyle habits [20, 21]. Yet, while contextual and lifestyle factors are more taken into account in the counselling process, patients and their families may still experience the fundamental and overwhelming question of 'Do I want to know?' in considering a test or while being confronted with the possibility of having a genetic disease.

This fundamental question also surfaced in the decision-making process of our interviewee: Mrs Alberta was overwhelmed by the confrontation with the unexpected knowledge and the fact that parts of her family had possessed this knowledge for a long time but had decided to keep it secret from the rest of the family.

Mrs Alberta's decision for taking a gene test is interpreted by us as her first step into a different pattern of action towards the disease. While the ethical perspective focuses on her need for security, the biographical analysis focuses on the freedom for acting as a consequence of her decision.

Some of the facets of the individual account presented in the analyses were only highlighted from a single interpretative perspective. These aspects are no less cogent as they result from the different focus on internal versus external structure. Instead, they complement each other and enable a broader view on the case study, providing a more complete analysis of the different aspects of the decision-making process. This allows the comparison of results that a single methodological approach by itself would not be able to yield.

The two complementary perspectives highlight the complexity of the radical change of behavioural patterns towards the disease: as the biographical analysis stresses, the separation of Mrs Alberta and her family originates with the decision of Mrs Alberta to not only deviate from the practices of her parental generation, but also to put a distance between her and her mother. The practice of not disclosing knowledge to other family members is from the ethical perspective interpreted as a problem of loyalty. This provokes a question: would the separation have happened in a similar way if Mrs Alberta's mother had proven her behaviour as more open to her daughter?

The biographical analysis shows that experiences from the past can be used by individuals to give structure to the present: Mrs Alberta refers to her mother's behaviour to define new own ways of acting differently. From the perspective of the biographical analysis, the decision is already laid out in the past; possible alternatives for action are thought through and weighted. The concrete decision itself can thus seem intuitive and spontaneous if we look at it just in the present. The biographical analysis further establishes Mrs Alberta's exposure to the unexpected genetic knowledge about Huntington's as a revelation and a central reference point for her interpretation of her biography and her future path of action. This suggests that the individual perception of events happening to the person at risk is central to the decision-making process. Every action that Mrs Alberta later commits herself to refers back to this moment of revelation, of perceiving a different order that provides a coherent argumentation structure.

In contrast, the second interpretative (ethical) perspective emphasizes the concrete present actions and those that commit them, e.g. it raises the question of responsibility and accountability: to what degree is Mrs Alberta's mother responsible for sharing the genetic knowledge with her children? And if she decides about the sharing, how are her daughter's resulting actions connected to her area of accountability? Normative focus is put on actual or hypothetical events originating from the different actors at stake.

In conclusion, we have shown how whole families are involved in the decision-making process and the keeping 'secret' or 'sharing' of genetic knowledge: While both methods present an a posteriori analysis of the biographical account, they each find complementing pieces of the puzzle. The biographical analysis follows the individual assessment inherent in the narrative and thus focuses on the perception of the individual and the resulting patterns that enable the individual to cope with and react to biographical events. The ethical analysis, in contrast, examines actions and their effects on others, and thus highlights existential individual questions.

Our results suggest a strong web of responsibility within at-risk families – strategies of coping with genetic knowledge will have to extend beyond the situation of the individual to include the interactions within the family. Similarly, genetic counselling should include the communication of genetic risk within the family [22]. In addition, cultural differences in the role of families have, for example, been demonstrated between the Netherlands and the US [23]. The history of not only individuals, but of all involved family members plays a defining role in the decision-making process. 'How will the life of others change? And how will that influence my own life?' become central questions for deciding what knowledge should be shared and what should be kept secret.

References

1 Swiss Academy of Medical Sciences: Genetische Untersuchungen im medizinischen Alltag. Basel, Swiss Academy of Medical Sciences (SAMW) 2004, p 9.

2 Burke W: Genetic testing. N Eng J Med 2003;347: 1867–1875.

3 Marteau T, Richards M (eds): The Troubled Helix. Cambridge, Cambridge University Press, 1996.

4 Chadwick R, Clarke A: Genetic counselling; in Chadwick R (ed): Encyclopedia of Applied Ethics, vol 2. London, Academic Press, 1998, pp 391–405.

5 Williams SJ, Birke L, Bendelow, GA (eds): Debating Biology. Sociological Reflections on Health, Medicine and Society. London, Routledge, 2003.

6 Smith JA, et al: Risk perception and decision-making processes in candidates for genetic testing for Huntington's disease: an interpretative phenomenological analysis. J Health Psychol 2002;7:131–144.

7 Scully JL, Porz R, Rehmann-Sutter C: 'You don't make genetic test decisions from one day to the next': using time to preserve moral space. Bioethics 2007;21:208–217.

8 Porz R, Widdershoven G: Predictive testing and existential absurdity: resonances between experiences around genetic diagnosis and the philosophy of Albert Camus. Bioethics 2011;25:342–350.

9 Krüger HH, Marotzki W (eds): Erziehungswissenschaftliche Biographieforschung. Opladen, 1994.

10 Schütze F: Kognitive Figuren des autobiographischen Stegreiferzählens; in Kohli M, Robert G (eds): Biographie und soziale Wirklichkeit. Stuttgart, 1984.

11 Smith JA: Interpretative phenomenological analysis; in Smith JA (ed): Qualitative Psychology. London, Sage, 2003, pp 51–80.

12 Etchegary H: Discovering the family history of Huntington disease (HD). J Genet Couns 2006; 15:105–117.

13 Van Riper M: Genetic testing and the family. J Midwifery Womens Health 2005;50:227–233.

14 Klitzman R, Thorne D, Williamson J, Chung W, Marder K: Disclosures of Huntington disease risk within families: patterns of decision-making and implications. Am J Med Genet A 2007;143A:1835–1849.

15 Porz R: The need for an ethics of kinship: decisions stories and patients' context; in Müller HJ, Rehmann-Sutter C (eds): Disclosure Dilemmas. London, Ashgate, 2009, pp 53–64.

16 Konrad M: Narrating the New Predictive Genetics. Ethics, Ethnography and Science. Cambridge, Cambridge University Press, 2005.

17 Rehmann-Sutter C, Porz R, Scully JL: Genetische Untersuchungen bei Kindern: Einige ethische Aspekte. Schweizerische Ärztezeitung 2004;51: 2787–2789.

18 Zwart H: De waarheid op de wand. Psychoanalyse van het weten (Dutch). Vantilt 2010; ISBN 9789460040481.

19 Kardorff E, Flick U, Steinke I: A Companion to Qualitative Research. London, Sage Publishing, 2004, pp 178–183.

20 Brand A: Public health and genetics – a dangerous combination? Eur J Public Health 2005;15:113–116.

21 Cecile A, Janssens JW, Khoury MJ: Predictive value of testing for multiple genetic variants in multifactorial diseases: implications for the discourse on ethical, legal and social issues. Ital J Public Health 2006;4:35–41.

22 Forrest LE, Delatycki MB, Curnow L, Skene L, Aitken M: Genetic health professionals and the communication of genetic information in families: practice during and after a genetic consultation. Am J Med Genet A 2010;152A:1458–1466.

23 Boenink M: Unambiguous test results or individual independence? The role of clients and families in predictive BRCA-testing in the Netherlands compared to the USA. Soc Sci Med 2010; Jun 25 [Epub ahead of print].

Dr. Rouven Porz
Ethics Unit, Executive Committee
Bern University Hospital 'Inselspital'
CH–3010 Bern (Switzerland)
Tel. +41 31 632 1956, E-Mail rouven.porz@insel.ch

Anne Brüninghaus, Dipl.-Päd.
Research Center for Biotechnology
Society and the Environment (BIOGUM)
University of Hamburg
DE–22529 Hamburg (Germany)
Tel. +49 40 7410 56310
E-Mail anne.brueninghaus@uni-hamburg.de

Ethical and Juridical Perspectives

Pfleiderer G, Battegay M, Lindpaintner K (eds): Knowing One's Medical Fate in Advance. Challenges for Diagnosis and Treatment, Philosophy, Ethics and Religion. Basel, Karger, 2012, pp 50–64

Predictive Medicine – Changes in Our View of Ourselves and Others

Dieter Birnbacher

Heinrich-Heine-Universität, Düsseldorf, Germany

Introduction

My points of departure are two platitudes about predictive medicine:

1 With the rapid progress of diagnostic technology, predictive medicine can be expected to go on expanding and to develop ever more extensive and more differentiated means of diagnosing genetically and non-genetically caused diseases and disease dispositions of a person, of his potential descendants and even of his living relatives.

2 This development is mainly beneficent, but at the same time, ambivalent. On the one hand, extending predictive diagnostics increases the chances of therapies and preventive measures that would not otherwise exist. Even if prevention by medical means is impossible, there are often ways of preventing, weakening or delaying the manifestations of symptoms by appropriate adaptive behaviour.

We know that an adaptive strategy can be highly successful. An instructive case of which I was made aware several years ago is the case of alpha-1-antitrypsine-deficiency in identical twins, a genetically caused disease which leads to the destruction of the elastic fibres of the lungs under certain conditions. One of the twins died of the disease at the age of forty due to smoking, whereas the other twin was still free of symptoms at the age of sixty.

On the other hand, we know that knowledge of one's own (and possibly some other person's) prognosis can mean heavy psychological strain. This is the rule, for example, in the well-known genetic disease of Chorea Huntington, a late-onset disease that can be prognosticated but neither prevented nor treated. Diagnosis and related information often means not only great psychological harm to the persons directly affected, but also to their non-affected relatives, for example, by the way of the phenomenon known as 'survivor's guilt'. Even with the lesser evils, knowing the (nearly) inevitable can plunge a person, and his or her near relatives, into desperation; knowledge of a mere risk-disposition can be highly problematic. Depending on the psychology of the person, it can trigger severe fear, anxiety and unrest. Self-knowledge is often a mixed blessing, and the ambivalence of it is well captured by the English word 'self-conscious': knowledge about oneself can be self-liberating, but it can also kill spontaneity and stifle the joy of existence. As we know also from breast cancer prevention strategies, diagnoses can cause heavy psychological damage, not least because diagnostic information is probabilistic and the untrained human capacity to process statistical information is severely limited.

What likely effects will this development have for our view of ourselves and others? I think that, as is usual in philosophy, the answer is complex. In particular, the answer depends what exactly is understood by 'our view of ourselves and others'. This can be understood in more than one sense, and the answer seems to depend on the preferred interpretation. One sense in which it can be understood is in a generic sense: will our view of ourselves and others in general change with the advances in predictive medicine? Another sense is the individual one: is our view of ourselves and others as individuals likely to change with the advances in predictive medicine?

The thesis that I want to defend is that the rapid progress of predictive medicine has not substantially changed our view of ourselves and others in general and can be expected to remain what it is. It has had, however, and will probably have, effects on our view of ourselves and others as individuals. The advances in predictive medicine do not seem to have changed substantially what has been called our general image of the species, our 'Menschenbild' (literal *German translation*: 'image of man'). However, these advances have the potential to change our view – and our dealings – with ourselves and others as individuals. This may result in new moral constellations and challenges for those who are in a position to access the relevant predictive medical information.

Ambiguities in the Concept of 'Menschenbild'

I hesitate to use the concept of 'Menschenbild' or the 'idea of man' because it seems to me that this concept is likely to cause confusion, which should be avoided. In particular, confusion is invited by the fact that this term is in many ways ambiguous and that its various meanings are not always separable.

There seem to be three principal ways or methods in which the concept of 'Menschenbild' is used in ethical, legal, and, in particular, theological debate:
1 descriptive,
2 hypothetical, and
3 evaluative/normative.

Each of these usages is rooted in specific contexts. In a *descriptive* sense, 'Menschenbilder' concepts purport to give an account of the constants of human nature. In a *hypothetical* sense, 'Menschenbilder' concepts suggest certain simplified patterns of human behaviour for purposes of theory construction, such as in game theory and economics (e.g. the *homo oeconomicus* model). In a *normative* sense, a 'Menschenbild' concept expresses a view of how humans ought be or behave, irrespective of how they in fact behave. Some of these categories can be subdivided, e.g. by distinguishing between *empirical* images of man, as they are discussed in psychology, and *speculative* images of man as they are discussed in theology. Analogously, a normative 'Menschenbild' can be meant as a *direct* norm (such as the much belaboured 'Menschenbild des Grundgesetzes' i.e. the concept of the basic laws that function as a normative premise of, among others, the social state) or as an *ideal* from which nothing in the way of obligations directly follows but which serves as an ideal reference point, for example, in education and educational policies (e.g. the 'Menschenbild of the Enlightenment').

Confusions arise if these necessary distinctions are neglected. There are quite a number of possibilities. One is *dogmatizing about human nature*, thereby ignoring the fact that our knowledge of man's nature is limited to the brief period of experience on which our conceptions are based and the vulnerability of constructions of 'human nature' to revision by new experience and changed conditions. In analogy to John Stuart Mill's point in support of female emancipation – that it is much too early to judge about the capacities of women from the experience of a historical period in which they were held in servitude most of the time – one should likewise warn against all prophets who reify 'human nature' as something constant and resistant to all future changes in social arrangements.

Another kind of 'pathological' case or confusion associated with the concept of 'Menschenbild' is that speculative images of man are described as if they were empirically based, whereas they are, in fact, idealisations or pious hopes. A case in point is Condorcet's 'Menschenbild' according to which man is wax in the hand of educators and is perfectible without limits. The extreme on the other end of the spectrum is the demonization of human nature by anthropological pessimists like Schopenhauer or Freud. Judging from mankind's record up to now, there is indeed little hope for optimism. But there are plenty of generations to come, and the books have not yet been closed.

A third confusion is taking for granted one's own *a priori* construction of human nature and drawing far-reaching normative conclusions from it. This has been a central issue in the discussion of contract theories in political philosophy from Hobbes to Rawls. The consequences these theories have for practical politics are reliable only to the extent to which the assumptions they make about human motivation are in conformity with reality. How far this is the case is, however, rarely examined. Obviously, this issue is a matter for empirical sciences such as psychology and sociology to decide and not for the armchair philosopher speculating about human nature.

Predictive Medicine and the Image of Man – Has Anything Changed?

We are now in a position to differentiate the question concerning the relation between predictive medicine and the 'image of man' and to focus on the question: has predictive medicine changed anything in the 'image of man' in a *descriptive* sense?

I do not see why this should be so. My argument is that there have always been ways by which one's health prospects were judged on the basis of a large and heterogeneous set of indicators. The prevalence of diseases in one's family has always been taken as indicators of medical dispositions and risks likely to materialize in the future. Parts of the traditional catalogues of vices, such as the doctrine of the deadly sins, offer themselves to a medical interpretation as warnings and admonitions about the fatal long-term consequences of gluttony, intemperance and debauchery. Of course, prognoses of long-term health were mostly based on general clinical and social experience instead of individual predictive tests. But this does not make any difference to the fact that man's destiny was always seen as partly predetermined by his bodily dispositions, both inborn and acquired. In particular, predictions of life expectancy were to a large extent possible on the basis of socio-economic factors. Even at the end of the 19th century, the average life expectancy of manual workers was no more than 67 years.

It is interesting to see that even then, medical predictions were not seen throughout as an inalterable 'fate'. They were often seen as challenges – by the persons concerned, by physicians, sometimes, also by a person's relatives. A poignant example is provided by the last weeks in the life of the German writer Theodor Storm, who wrote his most extensive novella, *Der Schimmelreiter* (*'The Rider on the White Horse'*), during a period of fatal illness in which he had been expected to be long dead. Storm's family concealed the true diagnosis from him by requesting the physician to perform a sham examination and to tell the author that the prognosis based on the first examination was wrong. In this way, Storm managed to muster the strength and discipline to complete the novella.

Nor is there any ground for thinking that predictive medicine has changed, and is likely to change, anything substantial in the *normative* image of man prevalent in our civilisation. It is widely admitted that the leading principles governing the dealings with individuals in medicine continue to be beneficence and autonomy. There is even evidence that the principle of patient autonomy will come to be seen as a principle that is at least as important as the principle of beneficence in parts of the world in which, nowadays, the more or less paternalistic conceptions of the doctor-patient relationship still prevail.

This is not to say that the consensus on these principles guarantees that there are no real ethical problems in dealing with predictive medicine. On the contrary, there are even now a great number of controversies about how these principles should be applied in concrete medical practice and about the weight that should be given to each of these principles in cases of conflict. This is particularly relevant to the present topic because in the practice of predictive medicine conflicts between these principles seem to be downright inevitable. These conflicts typically arise in the context of the *individual* patient and his and others' view of him.

What Has Changed – From the Viewpoint of Subjective Rationality?

It is highly probable that the advances of predictive medicine will change not our image of man in general but of ourselves as human individuals. Even if we do not make use of the tests that will be available in the future it is to be expected that our view of ourselves will be changed by the knowledge that such tests are available. At present, those who have their genes analyzed by the tests freely available on the Internet are mostly frustrated by the poorness of the information received. The information they receive is typically probabilistic and mostly irrelevant to possible preventive behaviour. However, the precision, the reliability and the breadth of the tests can be expected to increase considerably in the future as well as the capacity to establish connections between genetic data and disease dispositions. It is to be expected that this results not only in a purely quantitative increase, but, at a certain point, the quantity will be transformed into quality and we will begin to view our bodily condition and its prospects as something that can potentially be made radically transparent to ourselves and others.

From the point of view of subjective rationality, information about oneself and one's medical future is, however, a mixed blessing, for many reasons:

– because of the content of the information which may be more or less unpleasant,
– because the information subsumes me as an individual under a statistical class and does not respect my individuality,
– because of the innuendo of determinism associated with it, the real or apparent fact that there is nothing very much one can do about one's medical future.

I vividly remember an incident in my life that made keenly aware of the ambivalences of predictive medicine. When I had a sudden swoon during a medical examination following a bicycle accident, I was jokingly classified by the intern on duty as 'the type with cardiac infarct at retirement'. From the perspective of medical ethics, this verbal intervention was morally problematic in many respects: the jocular spirit on which it was uttered was inadequate to the context of a medical examination; it was an exploitation of an exceptional state of vulnerability; and, above all, it was involuntary and unwanted. (On the positive side, it might be said, the physician made use of an exceptional situation to get across a highly valuable warning.) From a moral point of view, the feature of voluntariness is certainly the crucial one. Even if a piece of information is accurate and sufficiently certain to be mentioned at all, being informed about one's medical future without consent clearly violates the patient's autonomy.

There are many reasons to insist on this autonomy:

1 We may not want to have this information because it means a burden that we simply do not want to bear.
2 We may not want to have this information because it is not rational, from the viewpoint of our own best interest, to have this information. Information can, for example, weaken spontaneity and the 'élan vital' or so-called vital impetus. Foreknowledge is generally welcomed, but not in an overdose.
3 We do not want to have this information because we do not want others to share this information and because we know that it will be difficult to keep it secret.

From the perspective of the patient, there are, then, compelling reasons to insist on a verdict of unwanted or otherwise involuntary information about his medical future, or, in other words, a right *not to know*. At the same time, he has good reasons to want to be able to refuse tests with potential predictive value that might be required in the context of seeking health or life insurance or in the context of employment, unless he can be certain that measures are taken that safeguard his right not to know without jeopardizing fairness in his relations with the insurance company (such as by delegating information about his health risks to his family doctor) or the legitimate interests of employers to minimize health risks on the job.

The patient's right not to know is one of the most uncontroversial tenets of medical ethics and has been firmly established by now by most legislatures. There remain, however, a number of constellations in which it is less clear that this right is paramount, for example, when others (such as partners or children) have an existential interest in knowing about the health status of a partner or relative, such as in cases of human immunodeficiency virus or of genetically related late-onset diseases.

Does Patient Autonomy Imply a Right to Know?

The more controversial issue in medical ethics in the context of predictive medicine is whether the patient has a *right to know* alongside with his *right not to know* and whether the physician is under an obligation to give the patient full information about his prognosis if he wants it.

In medical ethics, such an obligation is usually derived from the principle of *patient autonomy*. This derivation seems convincing at first sight, but is much less compelling when seen in the light of the fact that patient autonomy is usually interpreted as the right to *self-determination*. Can a right to self-determination be violated by a mere negative act such as the doctor not informing the patient about the intended or unintended results of a test? This is by no means evident, and especially so if the patient does not, for some reason or other, *ask* for these results. What we seem to have here is an ethical asymmetry between 'active' information and merely 'passive' non-information.

It is an important feature of the principle of patient autonomy that it imposes restrictions on *active* information, but that it does not seem to impose restrictions on *passive* non-information. The principle of autonomy directly entails a *right not to know* but it does not directly entail a corresponding *right to know*. If respecting the autonomy of a patient means not to do anything to him without his explicit or presumed consent, autonomy is a purely *negative* right, and the obligation to respect this autonomy a purely *negative* obligation.

Surely, this conclusion sounds paradoxical. After all, it is not at all unusual to base claims to being informed on the principle of autonomy.

The paradox dissolves when we take account of the fact that, again, the concept of autonomy is (as most fundamental concepts of ethics are) ambiguous. There are a number of clearly distinct meanings that have been arranged by the American legal philosopher Joel Feinberg [1] in the following instructive list:

1   autonomy as personal capacity,
2   autonomy as actual condition,
3   autonomy as ideal of character,
4   autonomy as a moral right.

This list is by no means complete. Philosophers will notice that more than one meaning of 'autonomy' is lacking, for example, freedom of the will, or moral freedom in the specifically Kantian sense. But the meanings distinguished by Feinberg are certainly the most important for practical purposes. Furthermore, Feinberg's list makes it evident that the concept of autonomy assumes quite a number of different semantic roles. In its first and second sense, autonomy is a descriptive concept, in its third and fourth sense, it is a normative concept. Again, these concepts are normative in different respects.

Autonomy as a moral right is something that can be claimed or enforced, whereas autonomy as an ideal of character is something that can only be recommended or made the basis of educational strategies. Autonomy as a moral right implies that others have an obligation to respect it, while autonomy as an ideal of character implies nothing of the kind.

Another distinction brought out by Feinberg's list is that between autonomy as a capacity (concepts 1–3) and autonomy as a claim (concept 4). Attributing one of these is logically independent from attributing the other. Saying that a person has a claim to autonomy does not imply that this person is autonomous. Saying that a person is autonomous does not imply that this person has a claim to autonomy. Even more importantly, saying that a person is not autonomous does not imply that the person has thereby forgone all claims to autonomy.

In the doctor-patient relationship, all four of Feinberg's concepts of autonomy have their particular role. Autonomy as a capacity is a condition of the ability to give consent, autonomy as an ideal functions as a regulative idea of the doctor-patient relationship, and autonomy as a moral right is an unquestioned normative criterion of all medical interventions except interventions in emergency situations.

That the ability to give valid consent is directly bound up with the patient's autonomy as a capacity seems to need no further comment. One should, however, say a word about patient autonomy as an ideal. This ideal, impressively described by the German psychiatrist-philosopher Karl Jaspers, is the ideal of a patient who is not only sufficiently autonomous to consent to diagnostic or therapeutic procedures proposed by the doctor, but who takes all medical decisions himself, the physician only providing the relevant information [2]. In this ideal, the customary role of doctor and patient are almost reversed. The judgement of what it is necessary to do is no longer the doctor's judgement, but the patient's. The role of the physician is reduced to giving a descriptive assessment of the prospects and risks of possible diagnostic and therapeutic measures which are then transformed into concrete directives by the patient, on the basis of his own personal values and preferences, including his risk preferences.

It is clear that this ideal of autonomy can at best serve as a regulative idea. Empirical investigations suggest that the great majority of patients have a preference for not getting involved in medical decision-making and the less so the more severe their disease [3]. At the same time, the reluctance of patients in this regard may just as well correspond to a genuine desire for not being bothered. Many medical decisions are difficult, especially if the diagnosis or prognosis is uncertain or a complex pattern of probabilities has to be taken into account. They would put a heavy strain on most patients even in their healthy days. This must be even more so under conditions of fear, depression and uncertainty which often accompany illness and disease. A further motive for patients not to get involved in medical decisions might be the desire not to interfere with the physician's own decisions, with the underlying (conscious or unconscious) thought that the physician might be more strongly motivated to help the patient if he can follow his own values and convictions instead of those of the patient.

One of the points of Feinberg's distinction is that the range of application of autonomy as a moral right to self-determination is considerably larger than that of autonomy as an ideal or as a durable or temporary capacity. It is clear that even those who do not, or do not want to, satisfy the conditions of autonomy as an ideal do not thereby lose their claim to self-determination. The same holds for autonomy in the sense of a capacity. Only if autonomy as a capacity is absent in a very fundamental sense, autonomy in the normative sense does no longer apply. Whoever is autonomous to such a slight degree that one cannot seriously talk of 'compulsion' or 'duress' in their regard is not a proper subject of a right to self-determination (e.g. babies, seriously demented people, etc.). But even those who are capable of self-determination only to a very limited extent do not thereby lose their right to self-determination. The fact that a person's will is essentially influenced by external factors is in general not sufficient to deny him the right to self-determination. The right not to be subjected to compulsion does not only apply to persons whose will is wholly or largely controlled by 'internal' rather than 'external' factors. The principle to respect the goals and values of a person does depend on the fact that a patient is able to make a choice. It does not depend on the degree to which this choice is free and autonomous.

Patient Autonomy as an Ideal

Though patient autonomy as a right is only weakly connected with patient autonomy as a capacity, it might, nevertheless, be asked if the doctor's task should not only consist in *respecting* the autonomy of his patient as a right but also to actively *further* the patients' autonomy as a capacity. In recent bioethical discussions, there has indeed been a tendency to suggest that the physician should not only respect his patients' wishes but should also educate his patients to become more competent, more responsible and more autonomous in their preferences [4].

However, a re-education of this kind is neither part of the principle of respecting autonomy nor of the ideal of individual autonomy characteristic of the Enlightenment tradition. An obligation to educate others by furthering their autonomy can be validly derived neither from the one nor from the other principle. Autonomy as a right does not imply any positive duty. Being a purely negative right, it can only imply negative duties. Even if taken as an ideal, it cannot impose any obligations. On the contrary, the question arises whether, or under which conditions, encouraging or educating patient autonomy is *permissible* in the first place. Whether it is permissible seems to depend on two conditions:

1 that making patients more autonomous is in their own interest (or in the urgent interest of third parties), and
2 that becoming more autonomous corresponds to these patients' autonomous will.

According to the first condition, educative efforts directed at furthering autonomy are permissible only if there are – in Brian Barry's terminology [5] – not only *ideal-regarding* but also *want-regarding* reasons for furthering autonomy, such as enabling the patient to make better decisions, either from the perspective of his enlightened self-interest or from the perspective of ethics.

According to the second condition, efforts at strengthening autonomy are themselves subject to the principle of autonomy, a fact of considerable importance especially in the practice of *psychotherapy* in which autonomy has traditionally been one of the dominant goals. Given the second condition, the psychotherapist is allowed to pursue goals of autonomy only to the extent fixed in the treatment contract. The patient must be able to rely on the fact that the therapist does not pursue other goals than those to which he has given consent, irrespective of the degree to which the therapist shares the patient's goals and preferences. However, this is not the only problem with autonomy as a goal of therapy. Another problem is that the goal of autonomy is only rarely stated explicitly. Autonomy is 'built into' psychotherapeutic methodologies such as psychoanalysis or humanistic psychology with the consequence that many psychotherapists are prevented by their professional loyalties to reflect on the goals which are inseparable from their method of choice. Against this, it must be insisted that the patient's right to self-determination can be violated by imposing autonomy goals on him no less than by imposing on him goals of adaptation. Even if the goal of developing autonomy is a 'matter of course' for most psychotherapists, it need not be for the patient. The patient might be more interested in goals opposed to autonomy such as emotional bonding, symbiosis or religiosity. Having these goals (and the values going with them) is not necessarily a symptom of limited autonomy, quite apart from the fact that the patient must not be deprived of the right to satisfy desires which, from the therapist's perspective, seem 'false', infantile or immature [6].

Which Principles Should Guide the Practice of Predictive Medical Information?

It should be clear that the principle of patient autonomy does not immediately imply an obligation on the doctor's part to inform the patient. If this is so, what other principles should guide this decision?

One possible strategy is to view the information about a predictive diagnosis as one of various kinds of medical interventions and to apply to it the same principles that are customarily applied to somatic and psychotherapeutic medical interventions. After all, 'informational interventions', as they might be called, are part of the physician's work no less than somatic ones and have no lesser impact on the patient.

Drawing on this analogy immediately yields a number of consequences. The first consequence is that the patient's wish not to be informed should, as a rule, be respected. He should not be informed against his will. Compulsory information would clearly violate the patient's 'informational autonomy'.

One should not conclude from this, however, that there must be an explicit informed consent for each individual act of information. As with somatic interventions, the preferences of a patient can be evident from what the doctor knows about the patient's general character and background. It would therefore be rash to call 'paternalistic' any act of information which is in the patient's best interest but which is given without explicit consent. An act of information (or, for that matter, of non-information) should be counted an act of paternalism only if it is *against* the patient's will. Of course, the safer strategy is to ask the patient for his explicit consent. But in many cases, this question will prejudge the general direction of the information and possibly frighten the patient. Who, after all, will ask a patient for his explicit consent to be informed if this information is thoroughly agreeable? In principle, nobody should be forced to know what he doesn't want to know, even if information is part of the presuppositions of an informed consent to a somatic intervention. As a rule, the patient must have the option not to be informed and to delegate the decision to the doctor.

A second consequence from the analogy of somatic and informational medical interventions is that the obligation to comply with a patient's wish to be informed is weaker than the obligation to comply with a patient's wish not to be informed. This consequence corresponds to the fact that the doctor's obligation to comply with a patient's wish for a certain medical intervention is generally weaker than his obligation to comply with a patient's wish not to be treated. There are a number of circumstances under which a doctor is usually held to be free *not* to comply with a patient's wish for treatment, e.g.:

1   if the treatment is harmful to the patient,
2   if the treatment does no harm, but no good either,
3   if the treatment is disproportionately costly (not only in monetary terms), or
4   if the doctor conscientiously objects to the treatment.

The first condition is particularly relevant to the information case. Information, even if desired by the patient, can do considerable harm. A bad prognosis can evoke panic, depression, or feelings of shame. Risk diagnoses can cause deep and lasting anxiety. In practice, one will attempt to mitigate deleterious consequences by offering psychological advice and care, or to make information depend on the provision of adequate collateral psychological treatment.

It might, nevertheless, be asked whether there is not, after all, a normative symmetry between giving and withholding information at least when *no* harm for the patient is imminent. Given that the risks for the patient are negligible, is not respecting the patient's right to know just as important as respecting his right not to know?

One might try to support this question by an argument analogous to one originally put forward by Sissela Bok [7]: If the patient does not want to be informed and the doctor informs him, the information is forced on him. If the patient wants to be informed and information is withheld, non-information is forced on him. In both cases, the patient is made to live differently from how he wants to live. If the principle of autonomy says that nobody should be forced to know more about himself than he wants to, does it not also say that nobody should be forced to know less about himself than he wants to?

In my view, the argument misconstrues the relation between non-information and compulsion. 'Compulsion' is only defined for positive action, not for non-action. Ignorance is nothing that can be 'forced' upon anyone. To say that non-information or non-disclosure 'forces' anything upon anyone is a highly misleading way of expression.

A much more promising argumentative route to a right to know starts from the concept of autonomy as a *capacity* instead of the concept of autonomy as a *moral right*: *Information is an essential precondition both of the exercise of the capacity of autonomy and of its development.* Though it may be doubted whether autonomy as a capacity is to be welcomed under all circumstances, it cannot be doubted that the exercise of autonomy is a good for everyone who possesses this capacity. Exercising autonomy for a rational control of present and future behaviour in the face of health risks is, however, dependent on truthful information. The autonomous patient needs to know about the dangers threatening him in order to adapt to these dangers using preventive measures, e.g. by eliminating or avoiding environmental factors triggering or reinforcing medical problems. Even in cases in which it is too late for prevention, as with terminal illness, the patient is dependent on truthful information in order to make use of his autonomy, if only in order to prepare for his impending death.

How strong is this argument for a right to know? It is as strong as the capacity for autonomy of the individual patient and his interest in exercising it. The argument is far from implying a right to know for all patients. It does, however, imply such a right for those who are capable of and have an interest in exercising this capacity. In contrast to the right not to know, the right to know is restricted in scope.

Provisional Conclusions

For practical purposes, we can draw four preliminary conclusions:
1 No information should be withheld from an autonomous patient whenever the patient wants the information, the information does not carry serious risks (e.g.

the risk of suicide), and the patient needs the information for a conscious and realistic life strategy.

2 The fact that a patient wants information need not be manifested by an explicit request. Often, it can be indirectly concluded from the patient's behaviour and character. The absence of an explicit request is not in every case indicative of an absence of interest in information.

3 Truthful information is important for the patient not only in the context of a medical intervention but also in other situations such as a terminal illness. Wherever a right to know exists, it is independent of whether the patient, if informed, would be able to do anything to prevent, weaken or delay the disease threatening him.

4 Withholding diagnostic and prognostic information from a patient who explicitly asks for it or otherwise signals that he is interested in it and who can be expected to cope with it, is justified only whenever active lying would also be justified. This seems to follow from the general consideration that, with the possible exception of the factor of intention, non-information is normatively equivalent to active lying. It is hard to see why 'passively' withholding the truth should be judged differently from active deception. Though a normative equivalence of doing and forbearing, commission and omission cannot be shown to hold for all kinds of behaviour (e.g. not for involuntary harms to life and limb, where doing is generally experienced as more threatening than non-doing [8]), this special factor plays no part in the contrast between active and passive deception.

There are, no doubt, situations in which a doctor is justified not only to withhold the truth but also to actively deceive a patient about his predictive diagnosis in order to avoid serious harm. Such a situation was reported some years ago in a case of Chorea Huntington running in the family. After the death of her mother-in-law, a mother deceived her two daughters (who were under age at that time) about the character of the disease from which their grandmother had died. She told them that the disease was not hereditary and that the daughters had nothing to fear from it. In this case, I agree with Günther Patzig's judgment [9] that lying was justified in order to allow the daughters to live a life free from anxiety. The obligation to tell the daughters arose, however, with their coming of age, when they were in fact informed by their mother about the heredity of their grandmother's disease.

Questions and Answers

Q. [*Manuel Battegay*]: It's more of a comment: I would like to challenge some of the terms. Information in clinics is very relative. I often see that younger doctors give much too much detail, for example, they give too much detail when patients don't want to know what the details are, for example, where the pathology lies. It is the 'truth', but if you go into detail, it can be brutal. They understood a long time ago that this was the case. It also can be the issue, where it is also relative, that many diseases are not diseases anymore in certain stages. I give the example of hypertension. Hypertension was a deadly disease only 60 years ago – Franklin Roosevelt was the best known example – he had a blood pressure of over 230 [mm Hg]. That was simple, the doctors had to inform him. Nowadays, we discuss what hypertension is, if it is above 120 or 130, certainly above 140, it is pathological? Should I inform someone about the consequences and about lifestyle [when patient is on the borderline] then?

These are very difficult situations. As doctors, this then becomes a legal issue. If we do not inform, then, most of us, and especially for those who have not been long in clinical practice, are afraid – that much later – if the patient has a stroke, the patient asks why didn't you tell me that a blood pressure of 135 is not as good as 125? It is extremely relative. The farther away time-wise we come from a disease, the easier it is not to inform; the closer we come, we become under pressure in many ways. We give the information before we even ask the patient what he even thinks about it. That is what I live with daily in visits when I consult on the wards.

A. [*Birnbacher*]: I think both of your questions are interesting but really different and carry a different weight. The first question is really problematic in medical practice. It is true that young doctors tend to give too many details that are rather frightening or unsettling for the patient. This is not justified and is not required according to recent regulations, which state that the information should be understandable and adapted to the level of the patient's capacity to understand it. This can be transcended in many cases, especially if the patient is not interested in the medical details and is more interested, as a rule, in the consequences that the diagnosis/prognosis has for his concrete life/lifestyle, or, for example, for his professional and personal life. This is of course something that the doctor cannot encompass, although he should be informed of such details. This is very important in chronic diseases, where the doctor plays a very different role, and has to consider how the chronic disease can be reconciled to fit in with the general life plan of the patient.

Q. [*Klaus Lindpaintner*]: If we take this concept of respecting the patients' right **not** to be informed to the next level, leaving legal issues and liability aside, could you envision that a patient would waive his right to be informed, and still agree to participate in a clinical research project? Informed consent means that it is essential that he signs the form and goes through the information process [by the doctor]. However, if he takes his autonomy to the extreme, to the point of saying 'I don't want to know about any of the implications of this research' or outcome but still wish to participate in the clinical research?

A. [*Birnbacher*]: Is the question 'Do you think that he can give up his right to informed consent'? To delegate or renounce his right? Informed consent is, as a rule, a requirement – a binding requirement – and the patient cannot be free to not make use of this right. Strictly, ethically, this is not out of the question. But, in fact, this is a very unadvisable policy to permit something like that because in this practical field, there must be certain fixed rules and clear obligations. I think in this case, informed consent is an essential, axiomatic precondition. The subject would not be allowed to

demand for certainty about the existence or absence of disease-related predispositions is also covered [6].

The *right not to know*, on the other hand, protects the self-determined and autonomous decision of the person concerned to abstain from taking notice of his or her genetic information, as well as the right not to be confronted with already available knowledge as to one's own genetic predisposition (for more details, see refs 6 and 11). Therefore, it constitutes an individual right to no longer learn more on oneself as one really wants to [6, 12]. This means that in a legally conducted genetic analysis the decision as to whether the findings will be acknowledged or not, must always be decided by the persons concerned. In addition, it should be noted that one's genetic information reveals information on genetically related family members, so that these findings likewise form important information about potential genetic disorders or family risk factors. These family members can always rely on their right not to know as well [2, 11].

Implementation on a Statutory Level: Federal Act on Genetic Testing in Humans

On a statutory level and with regard to genetic testing, the above described rights are implemented in the *Federal Act on Genetic Testing in Humans* (HGTA)[4]. In terms of genetic knowledge, the HGTA stresses, on the one hand, the importance of the right of self-determination (in the form of the right to know and the right not to know), the duty to professional secrecy and the compliance of data protection regulations. On the other hand, these rights are to be balanced and assessed, since the knowledge generated by predictive tests allows one to draw conclusions about the genetic constitution and medical risks of genetically related family members who were not directly involved in the genetic tests.

Disclosure of Genetic Data: Art. 19 HGTA

With Art. 19 of the HGTA, the Swiss legislator has opted to balance the interests involved according to the following principles:
   (a) *Disclosure to the person concerned*
   In perfect accordance with the outlined rights of informational self-determination, Art. 19 para. 1 HGTA stipulates that the physician may disclose genetic test results

---

[4] The Federal Act on Genetic Testing in Humans entered into force on April 1, 2007. The Act is applicable in the medical field as well as in the employment, insurance and liability sector and states under what conditions genetic testing in humans may be carried out. The Act aims to ensure the protection of human dignity and privacy. It further aims to prevent abusive genetic testings and use of data, to ensure the quality of genetic tests and the interpretation of their results. The Act is not applicable to genetic tests as part of research projects.

only to the person concerned or, if he or she is incapable of judgment, to his or her legal representative.

(b) *Expressly consented disclosure to family members, spouse or partner*

Under the condition that the person concerned has expressly consented to, the physician may disclose the test results to the person's family members, spouse or partner (Art. 19 para. 2 HGTA). In addition to the explicit consent of the person concerned, each disclosure of genetic test results by a physician is further conditioned upon a release from the duty of professional secrecy; this release is given by the person concerned.

Art. 19 para. 2 HGTA defines a group of people, in particular the person's relatives, spouse or partner, to whom the physician may disclose the genetic data; this list is not exhaustive [2, 10]. The person concerned may decide to make the genetic information available to even more or less people. In addition, also the extent of the information being disclosed can be determined by the person concerned and may, thus, be limited to just parts of it. For evidence reasons it is recommended to have all consent modalities in written form [2]. According to the Explanatory Report to the HGTA (*Botschaft*), the aim of this provision is, on the one hand, to enable therapeutic benefit for genetic relatives and, on the other hand, to provide non-genetically related family members (such as spouses or partners) with key information that may effect common family planning, and thirdly, to ensure the best support available for the family [10].

(c) *Disclosure to family members, spouse or partner without consent*

The most controversial provision is, however, contained in Art. 19 para. 3 HGTA. If the person concerned denies to consent to a disclosure of his or her genetic data, the physician may apply to the competent cantonal authority to be released from his or her duty of professional secrecy[5] should the protection of *overriding interests* of the person's family members, spouse or partner require that they receive this information. The cantonal authority may further request an opinion from the Expert Commission for Human Genetic Testing[6].

As already been pointed out, the disclosure of one's genetic information requires, as stipulated in Art. 119 para. 2 lit. f Federal Constitution, Art. 7 HGTA, Art. 321 and 321[bis] of the Swiss Criminal Code, the consent of the person concerned. The provision of Art. 19 para. 3 HGTA thus clearly differs from the set requirement and allows, on request and upon release of the duty of professional secrecy, the disclosure of test results to family members, spouse or partner by the physician without consent of the persons concerned. Prerequisite for the release of the duty of professional secrecy is an "overriding interest" of the said persons. Since this is a statutory exception to the consent requirement for information disclosure (as laid down in Art. 119 para. 2 lit. f Federal Constitution), the group of persons defined (family members, spouses and partners) is to be regarded as exhaustive [2]. The disclosure and handing

---

[5] As stipulated in Art. 321 para. 2 of the Swiss Criminal Code.

[6] Art. 19 para. 3 HGTA. For more details (in German) see: http://www.bag.admin.ch/themen/medizin/00683/02724/04638/index.html?lang=de

over of genetic information (without the sample) may not take place before the cantonal authorities have released the physician from the duty of professional secrecy. Moreover, as nothing is said about the fact whether the defined group of people must already maintain a doctor-patient relationship to the disclosing physician, it can be assumed that this is not a necessary requirement [2].

How the term "overriding interests" must be read and interpreted has been left open by the law; moreover, it is an indefinite legal term. The wording was adopted from the Data Protection Act (Art. 13) [10]; in addition, the Swiss Criminal Code also provides for a release of the duty of professional secrecy by taking into consideration divergent interests without specifying detailed criteria [10]. As in other situations, it will be necessary to decide on each case individually. Concretely, the competent authority is in charge of balancing the interests and of deciding whether the information interests of the family members, spouse or partner are rated higher than the privacy interests of the individual; if the answer is yes, then the physician will be released from his or her duty to professional secrecy. Thus, the Swiss legislative body has implemented quite an "elastic" interest balance formula that does not demand for a special situation of distress or a substantial overriding interest on the sides of the defined group of persons (see also 2, p 200 for further references). As far as it can be traced from the activity reports of the Expert Commission of Human Genetic Testing, no practical case has yet been reported.[7]

In order to examine in detail under what conditions overriding interests may be accepted, one has to differentiate between genetically and non-genetically related family members; spouse and partner belong to the latter. According to the Explanatory Report to the HGTA, overriding interests of genetically related family members may be acknowledged if they do not receive necessary therapeutic or prophylactic care—although this would be very important for them due to their genetic condition—and are therefore threatened by serious health problems [10]. What does this exactly mean? It means that an overriding information interest will be assumed if the disclosure of genetic information of the person concerned is essential to offer a genetically related family member at all necessary medical assistance [2].

If this medical assistance is, however, accessible without interfering into the data sovereignty of the person concerned, an overriding interest of the genetically related person has to be denied [2]. An overriding interest should further be denied if either no health care to medicate or to prevent the health deterioration is available at all; yet, genetically related family members are free to take a separate genetic test at their own request (see also 2, p 201). Moreover, it is assumed that no overriding interest is given if the probability of a disease predisposition of the tested person is only slightly higher than in the general population; to be of overriding interest it should require a greatly increased probability of negative health course [2]. However, one should keep

[7] For more details, see the "Activity Reports of the Expert Commission on Human Genetic Testing", 2007–2008 and 2009.

in mind, that—subject to exceptions—genetic test results are always only probability statements that do not allow for definitive conclusions about the genetic constitution of third parties [1, 3]. The question how much of the test results of the person concerned can at all be drawn to genetically related family members has, therefore, on request of the competent authority, to be answered by the Expert Commission on Human Genetic Testing [10].

An overriding interest of non-genetically related persons (such as the spouse or partner), can be recognised in the context of common family planning. It is assumed that this relates to situations in which the tested persons keep their (serious) genetic predisposition secret, although they are aware that the spouse/partner is worrying about familial genetic diseases and common children would have a high probability of being carriers of a serious genetic disorder [2].

Concluding Remarks

As stated above, the individual's right to informational self-determination and its two manifestations in form of the right to know and the right not to know are basically respected under Swiss law. Also the HGTA is committed to these rights, as it leaves the decision about the use and notice of the own genetic information to the persons concerned (Arts. 5, 6, 18 HGTA). In the HGTA, however, the right to informational self-determination is subjected to an assessment process as—under the existence of overriding interests—the disclosure of one's genetic information to a defined group of persons is declared legal although the person concerned has not consented to it.

This regulation allows for a feasible way to solve difficult conflicts of interests. Especially physicians are now able to file—either on their own initiative or on request of a family member—an application for release from the duty to professional secrecy in order to meet both their patients and the needs of their patient's family members. However, there are various concerns about the exception of the consent requirement. It is particularly questionable whether the described possibility of disclosing genetic information does, in fact, lead to an erosion of a family member's right not to know. What if family members don't even think of knowing whether they are at an increased genetic risk but the physician feels committed to inform them?

To what extent the non-consented disclosure of genetic information is justified, will always be decided on each case individually. However, the set interest balance formula of "overriding interests" is an indefinite legal term to which considerable legal uncertainty is inherent. The implementation of such an "elastic" interest balance formula namely bears the risk that a release from the duty of professional secrecy in favour of a third party and to the detriment of the right of informational self-determination of the person concerned may faster be justified than with a detailed set of applicable criteria. Because of this, however, special responsibility lies with the physicians as well as the competent cantonal authority, to apply and grant the release of the professional secrecy only in really legitimate cases. For the future and in practice, this requires the formation of precise reference points and their strict application (see also 2, p 204 for a similar conclusion).

Questions and Answers

Q. [*Dieter Birnbacher*]: I have a question concerning the practical consequences of the gene testing law in Switzerland on the background that it has striking similarities with the German law for the same purpose. One consequence seems to be that genetic counselling plays a more prominent role, for example, in the standard prenatal diagnosis undertaken by gynecologists. The practical consequence is that there is a significant lack of staff for these purposes, because the normal gynecologist is not trained as a genetic counsellor and must undergo additional training, which takes time, cost, etc. Are there any experiences in Switzerland, which I think had to introduce the same policy, with these practical dimensions of the new law?

A. [*Dörr*]: As in Germany, the Swiss Federal Act on Human Genetic Testing (HGTA) contains detailed rules for genetic counselling in the context of prenatal genetic tests (Art. 15 HGTA) and requires that medical doctors have received appropriate postgraduate training in order to prescribe genetic tests (Art. 13 HGTA). As far as I know no study has yet been published or is in progress to analyze whether the legal requirements set by the HGTA are complied with in practice. But experience with similar topics shows that practice, for various reasons, is not always as the law demands.

Q. [*Georg Pfleiderer*]: Could you comment on the general tendency or general attitude of the law concerning privatization of genetic information? It seems contraintuitive regarding the fact that genetic information is not really private concerning relatives for instance?

A. [*Dörr*]: Under Swiss law, the right to self-determination is one of the most fundamental rights. It gives each person the right to decide freely when, how, to whom and in which contexts personal and private information and especially genetic data will be disclosed. It is therefore up to the individual to decide what value he or she attaches to his/her own data. Especially the Swiss Federal Act on Human Genetic Testing provides a strong protection of the right to self-determination; this right is applicable in each phase of a genetic study in the medical field. Further, the Federal Constitution explicitly stipulates in Art. 119 para. 2 lit. f that genetic information is subject to the scope of the right to informational self-determination.

[*Pfleiderer*]: Yes, what about if, say, in a Huntington's family my sister insists on her right not to know? It affects me if someone else in my family knows it. I have no chance to ask her not to take the test.

[*Dörr*]: That is right. The right not to know protects the self-determined and autonomous decision of the person concerned to abstain from taking notice of his or her genetic information as well as the right not to be confronted with already available knowledge as to one's own genetic predisposition. This decision must be respected. And it is not only the person examined but everyone who has the right to refuse taking notice of the information about his or her own genetic heritage.

Q. [*Man N.N.*]: How about testing in children? Let us assume we have a mother with breast cancer, and she wants to know if the breast cancer antigen is present in her daughter? Can she force her daughter to be tested? Let's assume the daughter is fourteen.

A. [*Dörr*]: To answer your last question first: No, she can't force her daughter to be tested. It is a basic principle in the context of a medical treatment that a person, regardless of whether he or she is a minor or legally incapacitated, decides freely whether the treatment is carried out – provided he or she is capable of making a judgment. In a legal sense being capable of judgment (urteilsfähig) means that a person does not lack the ability to act rationally by virtue of being a minor or because of mental illness, mental incapacity, inebriation or similar circumstances (according to Art. 16 Swiss Civil Code). Deciding when a person is regarded as being capable of judgment is relative and always depends on the specific treatment in question. From a legal perspective, this is assumed if the person – in relation to the concrete medical treatment – possesses the required capacity of discernment as to its meaning and significance and decides about it. The capability of judgment of minors is taken as given if the child possesses the already mentioned skills by virtue of his or her mental and moral maturity. Although no fixed age limit is set, the capacity of judgment is regularly assumed at the age of 16. With regard to predictive genetic tests, however, the necessary capacity of judgment is taken as given at the age of 18 – due to the multiple implications and far-reaching information.

According to the Swiss Federal Act on Human Genetic Testing (HGTA) genetic tests may only be performed on individuals if they serve a medical purpose and the right to self-determination is ensured (Art. 10 para. 1). On a person incapable of judgment a genetic test may only be performed if the test is necessary to protect that person's health. Exceptionally, a test of this kind is permissible if there is no other way of identifying a severe hereditary disorder in the family or a corresponding predisposition and if the burden on the person concerned is minimal (Art. 10 para. 2).

[*Response from audience*]: In that case, I think it would not be necessary; it would be advisable not to do the test. Because the disease is not seen at this age, so the girl has enough time to wait and make a decision about this when she is a legal adult. But this is a special case.

Q. [*Klaus Lindpaintner*]: I would just like to mention that the American Society for Human Genetics has commented very clearly on that point. Unless there are immediate therapeutic consequences, no children under the age of being competent are to be tested and tests should be delayed until they can make their own decisions.

References

1 Deutsche Forschungsgemeinschaft: Prädiktive genetische Diagnostik. Wissenschaftliche Grundlagen, praktische Umsetzung und soziale Implementierung. Stellungnahme der Senatskommission für Grundsatzfragen der Genforschung, 2003, pp 16f, 22, 43. http://www.dfg.de/download/pdf/dfg_im_profil/reden_stellungnahmen/2003/praediktive_genetische_diagnostik.pdf (accessed May 12, 2011).

2 Rieder H: Genetische Untersuchungen und Persönlichkeitsrecht. Eine Auseinandersetzung mit dem Bundesgesetz über genetische Untersuchungen beim Menschen im medizinischen Bereich. Basel, Helbing Lichtenhahn, 2006, pp 1f, 198, 199, 200, 201, 204, 205ff.

3 Kollek R, Lemke T: Der medizinische Blick in die Zukunft. Gesellschaftliche Implikationen prädiktiver Gentests. Frankfurt, New York Campus, 2008, pp 17, 36ff, 41f, 44ff, 72ff, 234.

4 Müller JP, Schefer M: Grundrechte in der Schweiz. Bern, Stämpfli, 2008, pp 164ff, 167, 168f.

5 St. Galler Kommentar: Die schweizerische Bundesverfassung. Zürich, Dike/Schulthess, 2008, Art. 13 N 38, 40, 44.

6 Mund C: Grundrechtsschutz und genetische Informationen. Postnatale genetische Untersuchungen im Lichte des Grundrechtsschutzes unter besonderer Berücksichtigung genetischer Untersuchungen im Arbeits- und Versicherungsbereich. Basel, Helbing Lichtenhahn, 2005, pp 86ff, 93f, 106f, 107ff, 108f.

7 Rudin B: Die Erosion der informationellen Privatheit—oder: Rechtsetzung als Risiko?; in Sutter-Somm T, Hafner F, Schmid G, Seelmann K (eds): Risiko und Recht. Festgabe zum Schweizerischen Juristentag. Basel, Helbing Lichtenhahn, 2004, 415ff, 422ff.

8 Rhinow R: Grundzüge des Schweizerischen Verfassungsrechts. Basel, Helbing Lichtenhahn, 2003, § 14 N 1280.

9 Schweizer RJ: Privacy: Selbstbestimmung in der transparenten Gesellschaft; in Schweizer RJ, Burkert H, Gasser U (eds): Festschrift für Jean Nicolas Druey zum 65. Geburtstag. Zürich, Schulthess, 2002, pp 907ff, 920.

10 Botschaft zum Bundesgesetz über genetische Untersuchungen beim Menschen (GUMG) vom 11. September 2002 (Explanatory Report HGTA). BBl 2002, pp 7361ff, 7398, 7422f.

11 Dörr BS: Blut, Gewebe, Zellen, DNA und Daten—Biobanken im Spannungsfeld von Persönlichkeitsrechten und Forschungsvisionen; in Dörr BS, Michel M (ed): Biomedizinrecht. Entwicklungen Perspektiven Herausforderungen. Zürich, Dike, 2007, pp 443ff, 464.

12 Hausheer H: DNS-Analyse und Recht: Eine Auslegeordnung. ZBJV 128, 1992, pp 493ff, 511.

Dr. Bianka S. Dörr, LL.M.
University of Zurich
Faculty of Law
CH–8001 Zurich (Switzerland)
Tel. +41 44 634 41 78, E-Mail Bianka.Doerr@rwi.uzh.ch

Religious Perspectives

Pfleiderer G, Battegay M, Lindpaintner K (eds): Knowing One's Medical Fate in Advance. Challenges for Diagnosis and Treatment, Philosophy, Ethics and Religion. Basel, Karger, 2012, pp 74–86

Fate and Judaism – Philosophical and Clinical Aspects

Benjamin Gesundheit

Department of Jewish Philosophy, Hebrew University, Jerusalem, Israel

Introduction: Medical Ethics and Jewish Medical Ethics

In a world and a field where there are so many subspecialties, it is particularly important to build bridges between disciplines. Historically, Basel has a great tradition of building bridges, and therefore, it is quite appropriate to talk here in Basel about bridges between medicine and ethics. Furthermore, KARGER Publishers has served as a most important bridge in this context, for it was KARGER who in 1911 published the milestone work in Jewish medical ethics – Julius Preuss' (1861–1913) masterpiece, "*Biblisch-talmudische Medizin: Beiträge zur Geschichte der Heilkunde und der Kultur überhaupt*" [1].

In order to build bridges between clinical medicine and medical ethics, we must learn from each other. We are not treating diseases, we are treating human beings, and therefore, we must understand their cultures, their belief systems and their personalities. Comparing cultures and intercultural approaches is extremely important for ethical discussions, as elaborated by Jürgen Habermas as the concept of "the ethics of discussion" [2]. My goal here is to present aspects of Jewish medical ethics, from which I trust we can derive certain clinical applications.

A hundred years ago, Sir William Osler (1849–1919) pointed out the importance of a **broad** general education for physicians. When physicians treat patients, they have to understand them in the context of their cultural background; in order for doctors to provide optimal patient-oriented treatment, medical humanities must be a component in their medical education. Medical humanities as a new medical adventure is presented in several recent papers [3, 4]. It is my hope that clinical ethics will be introduced into medical training programs and become an integral part of medical schooling. Personally, I work on the Hebrew website www.jewishmedicalethics. org which hopefully will soon be translated into English. I intend to present Jewish

Medical Ethics in a systematic manner, divided into the following three sections: (1) principles and basic concepts of ethics in Jewish tradition; (2) the role of medicine, the patient, the physician and the health system; and (3) practical questions following the human life-cycle (which is by far the largest of the three sections). Theoretical background material and classical sources will be presented in order to extrapolate from them practical and applied concepts for clinical medicine.

Jewish medical ethics has certain unique features. It is based on one of the oldest and most longstanding traditions in human history, going back to the Bible, the classical rabbinical sources in the Mishna and the Talmud, and the Responsa literature which continues until today. The exploration of these topics is extremely important: on the one hand, it requires a careful study of the classical sources, and on the other hand, it demands an understanding of contemporary issues and the challenges posed by recent developments. This continuous process creates the corpus of Jewish law which is called in Hebrew *Halakha*. The literal meaning of this term is "going" or "flowing", as all the sources of Jewish Tradition continuously "come to us" from Biblical times to our days.

Fate and Judaism

I shall open with a discussion of some of the purely religious and philosophical aspects of the issue. Afterwards, I shall present some clinical aspects and practical considerations.

A. Philosophical Aspects: The Permission and the Duty to Heal

There is an interesting philosophical question whether human beings are permitted and perhaps even obligated to engage in medical research and practice [5] This presentation of a Talmudic source, together with its medieval commentaries and its modern analysis by Rabbi A.Y. Kook will introduce the reader to certain basic philosophical concepts as well as to Talmudic thinking.

The Talmudic Source
We find in the Talmud – written about 1,600 years ago – an interesting text dealing with the permission granted by the Torah to heal and to be healed (in the context of the ancient custom of blood-letting). Two contradictory opinions are put forward by rabbinical scholars of the 4th century CE, reflecting two different philosophical attitudes:

*"As **Rav Acha** said: When going in for blood-letting, one should say: 'May it be Your Will, O Lord my God, that this operation may be a cure for me, , and may You heal me,*

for You are a faithful healing God, and Your healing is true,' since men have no power to heal, but this is the common practice."

According to this first approach, only God is the real Healer; the physician must justify his role and apologize for interfering with God's governance of the world.

Abaye presents another approach:

*Abaye said: People should not say this, because it was, taught in the House of Rabbi Yishma'el, 'And **he shall** certainly **heal**' (Exodus 21:18) – from here [we derive] that the physician is given permission to heal.*

The Biblical proof text suggests that engaging in the healing process is not only a theologically permitted activity, but even a religious duty that falls upon the physician. According to this second approach, a doctor has no need to apologize, as his role is fully justified.

Four Medieval Commentaries on this Talmudic Source
This Talmudic debate of the 4th century, whether or not a person should heal or accept medical help, continues in the later rabbinical literature, where four medieval commentators offer four different opinions regarding this Talmudic disagreement. Each of the four rabbis tries to explain the assumption why medical practice might need special "permission," why one might have thought that it is forbidden. These explanations provide additional insights into the Talmudic source:

1 *Rabbi Yaakov of Orleans* (died in 1189) suggests that theoretically a doctor should always heal for free, based on the Biblical commandment of "You shall love your neighbor as yourself" (Lev. 19:18). One should heal freely, out of love. However, since physicians obviously need to make a living, the Torah grants a physician permission to accept payment for his services.

2 *Rabbi Moshe ben Nachman, Nachmanides* (1235–1304), himself a practicing physician, recognizes the risk-benefit ratio in every medical procedure and that the physician must not cause any damage to his patient ("*primum nihil nocere*"). Therefore, considering the potential risk of medical treatment, the Torah must indeed provide explicit "permission" to heal. Once the physician carefully assesses the risks and potential adverse effects of his treatment, he has full "permission" to proceed, and actually fulfills the religious duty to heal.

3 *Rabbi Shlomo ben Aderet, Rashba (1235–1310)*, concerned in his generation with external cultural influences on Jewish tradition, states that the study and practice of medicine are certainly not violations of religious tradition, since the Torah grants explicit "permission" to heal. According to this explanation, one is allowed to study medicine in the same manner as one studies Biblical and other religious sources; medicine is accepted and considered as a religious science.

4 *Rashi* (1040–1104) and *Tosafot* (12th-14th century) relate to the theological diffi-
culties relating to medicine. They emphasize that medicine does not conflict with
Jewish theology. Therefore, a patient seeking medical help does not challenge
Divine providence in any way, for the Bible gives full "permission" to heal.
Furthermore, a sick person is not allowed to reject medical treatment, saying he
does so out of deference to God who made him ill.

Each of these four opinions presents a different understanding of the "permission"
that was granted to engage in medical practice; each of these rabbinical authors elabo-
rates on a different aspect of the obligation to heal. We do not find any accepted view
supporting a prohibition to study medicine and heal.

Rabbi A.Y. Kook's Interpretation: Synthesis of Classical Sources with the Modern Challenges of Medicine in the 20th century

Rabbi Avraham Yitzchak Kook (1865–1935) – one of the most illustrious figures in
Jewish philosophy in recent generations – dealt with the challenges that modernity
and social philosophy posed to Jewish tradition. He worked toward a synthesis of classic religious tradition and modernity, including science and medicine. Rabbi Kook's
writings demonstrate that he was fully aware of the challenges of modern medicine
and had a deep insight into psychology and psychosomatics.

Rabbi Kook interpreted the four medieval rabbinical explanations of the Talmudic
source in a most innovative way. He gave new meaning to each explanation:

1 According to R. Kook, monetary remuneration of a physician brings medicine
down to a level lower than that intended by the Bible. Ideally, medicine should
be practiced out of love for one's fellow man and not for any ulterior motives.
Since, however, a physician also has to make a living, he is permitted to heal in
exchange for money. Only God heals solely out of love and His healing succeeds
because it is directed at both man's body and his soul. Rabbi Kook's "upgraded"
explanation provides us with a deeper understanding of Rabbi Yaakov of Orleans'
viewpoint.
2 Nachmanides recognized the risk-benefit ratio. Rabbi Kook goes even further,
explaining that we are dealing with a delicate balance between body and soul.
The physician never knows in advance how a specific treatment might affect
another part of the patient's body or his psychological well-being, and therefore,
the physician might inadvertently cause damage in particular regarding the balance of body and soul. According to Nachmanides, a physician should not be
deterred by these risks; as long as he is cautious, he is permitted and even obligated to heal.
3 Rashba maintains that the study of medicine is a religious activity and that a physician fulfills a religious duty, as God wants human beings to understand the created
world and the science of medicine as an integral part of that world. The spiritual
world of Jewish religious studies versus the academic research of natural sciences
and medicine needs to be in a proper balance.

4 Rashi and Tosafot emphasize that one should not think that only God is permitted to heal, and that a doctor only interferes with Divine providence. Man is duty bound to improve the world; wisdom will help the wise man, and advances in human wisdom are all the work of God which becomes revealed in accordance with the needs of man in each area and every generation. A person has to carefully find the balance between his trust in God and his own proactive behavior to achieve God's blessings.

Rabbi Kook's analysis of the four classical medieval explanations of the Talmudic text provides new insights and upgrades the Talmudic discussion in light of the challenges of modern medicine at the beginning of the 20th century. Rabbi Kook emphasizes important modern insights into the body-soul relationship. Medicine does not interfere with Divine providence or religious values, as the physician fulfills God's mission to improve the world and help sick people in need.

Conclusions regarding "Knowing One's Medical Fate in Advance"

It would be wrong to think that according to classical Jewish tradition, one must accept fate and not interfere with Divine providence. Since man has been granted permission to heal and he is obligated to improve the world, he must not adopt a passive role for wrong religious concepts; on the contrary, he must be proactive and offer healing without hesitation, as the Bible and the Talmud encourage and support healing.

Rabbi Kook emphasizes that the practice of medicine is a Divine obligation – in full keeping with Divine providence – and its goal is to improve the world.

B. Clinical Aspects

How do these principles of Jewish medical ethics translate into practical clinical guidelines regarding "***Knowing One's Medical Fate in Advance***"? The Bible and the Talmud certainly knew nothing about modern technologies, such as genetic testing and prenatal diagnosis, and the related ethical questions. However, surprising as it may seem, the Talmudic literature is rich in sources that are relevant to these modern questions.

In order to address the central question of our conference as to the question to which extent knowledge should be shared, I wish to discuss certain relevant sources regarding abortion, prenatal testing and truth telling. In *Halakha*, the Jewish law, common sense is essential and contradictory sources can often be reconciled. What is more, contradictory messages arising from the Talmudic sources often accurately reflect contradictory situations in real life. I will, therefore, try to identify the contradictory messages of several Talmudic sources in order to better understand the logic behind them.

Abortion

The Mishna *Ohalot* 7:6 discusses the indications to perform an abortion. The topic being vast, I would like to focus on the specific aspect of embryotomy with respect to the question of knowing one's fate in advance:

"If a woman is undergoing difficult labor, one cuts up the child [fetus] in her womb and brings it forth member by member, because her life comes before that [of the child]. But if the greater part of the fetus has proceeded forth, one may not touch it, for one may not set aside one person's soul for that of another."

If an unborn fetus endangers its mother's life, and it is unlikely that both mother and baby will survive, an embryotomy must be performed in order to save the mother's life. However, once the head has passed through the narrow birth channel, one must not harm the baby in any way, because one soul (the child's) may not be set aside for another (the mother's).

In the Mishna, the relationship between mother, baby and fetus is clearly defined. The first section of the Mishna speaks of "life," while the latter section deals with the "soul." In'soul'ment takes place only with birth; prior to birth, the fetus is defined as "life," based biologically on heartbeat and other criteria of "life." Once the baby is born and starts breathing on its own, the newborn acquires the status of a "soul" like its mother.

It may be concluded from the Mishna that a fetus' life must be destroyed if it presents a direct birth-related danger to the mother. An interesting and most relevant question arises what to do when we know that the newborn's life will be in mortal danger immediately after birth or shortly thereafter, e.g., when there is a prenatal diagnosis of Tay-Sachs disease, severe heart malfunction, or another life-threatening neonatal condition that is not compatible with life.

Modern responsa literature provides a tragic example. In 1942 during the Holocaust period, a pregnant woman living in the Kovno ghetto and about to be deported to Auschwitz asked her rabbi whether she should perform an abortion, knowing that a pregnant woman could not possibly survive the Nazi selection process. Does the knowledge of a tragic fate in the very near future justify performing an abortion now? Rabbi Ephraim Oshry [1914–2003], the rabbi in the Kovno Ghetto, instructed the mother to abort even though there was no direct birth-related danger. He argued that it is not the mechanical process of giving birth which justifies abortion but rather her fate in the very near future. Rabbi Ephraim Oshry survived the war and published his responsa in the late 1960s in New York. [6] His halakhic decision demonstrates that abortion is indicated not only in the presence of a direct birth-related danger to the mother, but also if the danger to the mother is based on clear knowledge of her fate in the near future.

What is Halakha's approach to severe neonatal conditions such as the genetic disease Tays-Sachs, serious infectious complications (such as syphilis, toxoplasmosis, rubella, cytomegalovirus, herpes simplex [STORCH] or others) or chemotherapy

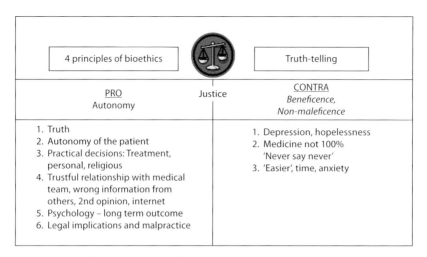

4 principles of bioethics		Truth-telling
PRO Autonomy	Justice	CONTRA Beneficence, Non-maleficence
1. Truth 2. Autonomy of the patient 3. Practical decisions: Treatment, personal, religious 4. Trustful relationship with medical team, wrong information from others, 2nd opinion, internet 5. Psychology – long term outcome 6. Legal implications and malpractice		1. Depression, hopelessness 2. Medicine not 100% 'Never say never' 3. 'Easier', time, anxiety

Fig. 1. Truth-telling according to the 4 principles of bioethics.

given to the mother during pregnancy? Are these indications for abortion as well? These questions open important and interesting discussions, and there are various and even contradictory opinions in the modern responsa literature, based primarily on the mother's personal attitude, the stage of pregnancy, and many other factors.

When I was in medical school and first developed an interest in these topics of Jewish medical ethics, I sought clear-cut guidelines for each case. It took me some time to fully appreciate the rabbinic approach which assesses the situation at hand on a case-by-case basis in order to provide a sensitive and balanced decision. As accurately articulated by my Talmud teacher, Rabbi Dr. Aharon Lichtenstein [7]: *"The question of abortion involves areas in which the halakhic details are not clearly fleshed out in the Talmud and Rishonim, and in addition, the personal circumstances are often complex and perplexing. In such areas there is room and, in my opinion, an obligation for a measure of flexibility."*

Before deciding about a particular case, one must carefully assess the situation in a sensitive and responsible manner: What does the abortion mean for the mother? One must ask her this question, discuss the matter with her and share one's thoughts with her. It is a joint decision which takes the mother's feelings into consideration.

Truth Telling and the Patient-Physician-Relationship
First, let us look at the theoretical concepts underlying the pros & cons of truth telling (Fig. 1). Without a doubt, telling the truth needs no justification, as speaking the truth is a value in itself. We must respect the autonomy of the patient regarding practical decisions. It is our goal that the patient develops a trusting relationship with his medical team and not receive relevant medical information from other sources.

The notion that by withholding the truth, the caretaker somehow makes it 'easier', saves time, or lessens anxiety is mistaken and has been proven wrong [8]. On the other hand, the patient might experience depression and a feeling of hopelessness when bluntly faced with the truth. The question, then, is how to integrate autonomy and the concept of beneficence, and thus do justice to our patients.

Halakhic literature is rich in sources dealing with telling the truth, three of which I would like to share with you.

First of all, the Talmud states that God's signet is truth (*Sanhedrin* 64a). This does not really need an explanation. Elsewhere (*Shabbat* 10a) the Talmud says:

"Any judge who renders a true judgment 'to its truth' even for one hour, Scripture considers him as though he had become a partner to the Holy One, blessed be He, in the creation."

What do the words, "a true judgment *to its truth*," mean? The commentators explain that an absolute truth exists, but it is difficult for us to discern it, as the absolute truth is not always evident. But each patient and each situation has its own context and its own truth. As judges or physicians, we have to understand and feel what is true for our patient now, in his particular situation, and at this particular moment. We also have to recognize that it might change over time or be different for each patient.

According to Jewish tradition, many blessings are recited over a variety of things and events. For example, upon seeing a great mass of people, one must recite the blessing: *'Blessed are you. . . that discerns secrets'* (*Berakhot* 58b). Upon seeing many different people, one must be careful not to generalize, but rather to look out for the individual human being, his needs and wishes. Each person is different in appearance, has his own mind, personality and secrets, and feels and thinks differently. This idea must always be kept in mind. This blessing guards us against generalization and oversimplification.

This reminds me of Emanuel's [9] famous paper in medical ethics where he describes four models in the relationship between the physician and his patient. He provides a useful guideline for understanding the patient, summarized succinctly in the rule that a physician must 'foresee' (="4C") his patient. The four C's are: **C**ure, **C**are, **C**ope, and **C**omfort, meaning that at different stages, the physician has to cure, care, cope or comfort his patient – all in accordance with the patient's needs at the time. This is one of the special challenges of clinical practice.

Maimonides, the famous Jewish philosopher, rabbi and physician, [10] stated this idea very clearly: *'Don't treat the disease, treat the patient'*. One of his patients said of him:

"Galen's art heals only the body, but Abu-Amran's (Maimonides') body and soul. His knowledge made him the physician of the century. He could heal with his wisdom the sickness of ignorance."

Let me mention here a unique and very interesting medical letter by Maimonides to his patient, the Sultan, who suffered from depression [10]. Since no anti-depressant medications were available at the time, Maimonides suggested that the Sultan should consider drinking alcohol, even though as a Muslim he is forbidden to do so. In his letter, Maimonides displays the concept of informed consent and leaves the final decision to his patient. Furthermore, at the beginning of his letter Maimonides cites from the Koran (4:79–81), thus showing his patient that he understands and appreciates his belief system. It was as if Maimonides were telling him that he must find a responsible balance between the appropriate medical treatment of depression and the religious prohibition of alcohol.

The Bible (Genesis 18:12–13) provides us with another example of truth telling when Abraham and Sarah are informed by God at the respective ages of 100 and 90 that they will have a baby.

"So Sarah laughed to herself, saying, 'After I am grown old, shall I have pleasure, my lord being old also!' And the Lord said to Abraham, 'Why did Sarah laugh, saying, 'Shall I indeed bear a child, though I am old?' "

Upon careful reading, one notices that God introduced a subtle change in the wording of Sarah's statement: Sarah had said that **Abraham** was too old to have a child, but God told Abraham that Sarah had complained that it was **she** who was too old to give birth. It is clear that God changed the wording in order to maintain a peaceful relationship between the couple. The Talmud (*Yevamot* 65b) teaches: *"One may modify a statement in the interests of peace. . . Rabbi Natan said: It is a religious obligation.* At the school of Rabbi Yishmael it was taught: *Great is the cause of peace, seeing that for its sake even the Holy One, blessed be He, modified a statement; for at first it is written* (Genesis 18:12): *'My lord being old,' while afterwards it is written (ibid. 14): 'Though I am old.' "*

According to the Talmud, it is permitted and even religiously mandatory to deviate from the truth in a matter that would disturb the peace if the truth were told. When telling the truth, one must be exceedingly sensitive and find a way to get the information across without hurting anybody's feelings. One must learn the psychological skills to communicate in a sensitive and subtle manner; the necessary adjustments are not considered lying, since the main issues are presented truthfully.

Another interesting and important Talmudic source regarding truth telling relates to the laws of mourning the death of a family member. The Talmud (*Mo'ed Katan* 26b) instructs us not to inform a sick person about the death of a family member if this information is likely to endanger his health or well-being:

"An ill person whose relative died, they should not inform him thereof, lest he become distracted in mind; nor do they direct to have any garments rent in his presence, and they direct the women to keep silent [from lamenting] in his presence."

Although the patient has the 'right to know' and, in the Talmudic context, also a religious obligation to observe the rites of mourning, one is obligated to protect him and not cause his mind to become distracted ("break his heart") or endanger his health. At times, the physician must show preference to the patient's beneficence, according to his own assessment, over the patient's "unlimited" autonomy if this would threaten his well-being. In order to protect the patient, the truth must sometimes be withheld.

Let us close with a more positive example from the Talmud regarding praising the bride at a wedding (*Ketubot* 16b–17a):

"How does one dance before the bride? **Bet Shamai** *say: [We praise] the bride as she is.* **Bet Hillel** *say: [In all cases we say] "A beautiful and graceful bride". Bet Shamai said to Bet Hillel: If she was lame or blind, does one say about her: "A beautiful and graceful bride"? The Torah says: "Keep yourself far from falsehood" (Exodus 23,7).*

Bet Hillel said to Bet Shamai: According to your words, if one has made a bad purchase in the market, should one praise it in [the purchaser's] eyes or depreciate it? Surely one should praise it in his eyes."

The Sages learned from this that *"a person's disposition should always be pleasant with people,"* meaning that one should always try to understand his fellow man's subjective truth. It might be better not to say aloud what one really thinks. Even if the truth is a subjective truth, the new couple's happiness is – on the halakhic level – more important than the objective, so-called absolute truth. The couple is looking forward to their shared future. The bride is beautiful in her groom's eyes, regardless of whether she is objectively so. The truth is presented in a way that is good for them. In this case, we do not deviate from the truth but present it in a positive way following the subjective truth of the people involved.

When thinking about knowing one's fate in advance, let us keep in mind the English notion of 'looking forward'; one must adopt a positive and optimistic attitude that respects the subjective perspective of the person involved.

Summary

There is a basic obligation – philosophically and theologically – to know, study, discover and improve the world, and, therefore, we have been granted the permission and given the duty to advance medical progress. On the practical level, a sensitive way must be found to convey bad news without causing emotional or physical harm; communication skills are crucial in order to recognize and respect the subjective feelings and the practical relevance of knowing one's fate in advance. If knowing one's medical fate in advance has practical relevance, this information should certainly be shared; however, beneficence remains the overriding principle and outweighs the patient's autonomy ('right to know'). The patient's subjective psychological wellbeing must be recognized and respected; withholding the truth or presenting it with special communication skills and in the most sensitive manner is essential.

Questions and Answers

Q. [*Regine Kollek*]: Is the notion of subjective truth true everywhere in Jewish society? For example, in the case of a crime, the person who committed the crime might – subjectively – think that he has a good reason for doing it. Would that be acceptable according to Jewish law?

A. [*Gesundheit*]: Certainly not. A crime is a crime, and the Law has very clear definitions and guidelines. I was talking about interpersonal reactions and information. [Fields of forensic questions, and mental diseases, is what he had in mind, of course that is not subjective truth. If he is sick, that is one thing, but he cannot just claim it like that.]

Q. [*Peter Sebastian*]: Did I understand the statement about Rav Kook correctly? Did he not contradict himself with the first statement from Ishmael about not taking money for the services?

A. [*Gesundheit*]: According to one opinion, the reason why you *might* think you should **not** perform medicine is because you have to take money. That might be a reason not to go into medicine, since one would have to work for free! Meaning, all physicians would work day and night, including weekends and night calls for free, since one should do it out of love. So, **the permission** is that one is allowed to take salary. [This is an interesting concept and the technical aspects or financial aspects: this means they can violate the beauty of medicine – which is basically out of love. God does it out of love, but you do it for free. That is the concept.]

Q. [*Jens Schlieter*]: Do you think that the difference between religion and philosophy could be described thus: the philosophical sources are in a constant process of renewing and adapting to the modern world, whereas the religious sources are essentially the same? Do you think of any possible new biomedical inventions that would put stress on the religious sources in a way that they would not be able to answer the ethical impact?

A. [*Gesundheit*]: This is a very interesting question. There are classical, philosophical and theoretical sources which are applied in a modern way. The interpretation, in my opinion, is a challenge for Jewish medical ethics. Take all the sources, read them, understand them, identify how they are working and apply them. Is this really new? Is this the new literature or the old one that continues?

I wanted to show this with the question of abortion. The concepts are old. But the mind has new wheels and it moves on. The concepts of abortion: when is it allowed, is it a direct danger, an indirect danger, a possible potential danger? These are legal questions which the skilled individual who is versed in the Jewish sources can apply.

In my opinion, this is the beauty of it: you can apply the old Jewish sources to the new developing questions. To do this, one needs skills which is the interesting part!

Q. [*Manuel Battegay*]: A lot of the Jewish ethics entered the mainstream in the early 20th century, keeping in mind that 50% of university physicians in Vienna and Berlin before the Second World War were Jewish. So I think a lot was brought into the mainstream. How is that now in Israel? How does it work daily? For less religious physicians? You have ethical consultancy, you give lectures in Tel Aviv and Jerusalem, so how is that compared with daily practice? Are you asked daily about religious laws, also by Orthodox people, who want to know, in view of new treatments, where they are insecure?

A. [*Gesundheit*]: This is also a very interesting question. The population in Israel is extremely heterogeneous. You have people who come from different religious backgrounds so they want to know if they can continue their previous activities and see how it fits in with the law. There are others who are definitely not interested and are anti-religious. There are people who I have the honor to present at Grand Rounds – Arabs. I enjoy talking to them very much. They say 'I like Rav Kook he's the best' and they start to argue with me about the sources that are inside. So all colors are there. So, summarizing what was said earlier today – you don't have to accept them as Law – if somebody wants it fine, if they don't, that's fine too. They are just very interesting sources: how to represent truth, how do I define truth? I hope that these sources can help the physician to make up his mind.

Q. [*Mr. Joshi, Hindu Scientist*]: I would like to add two small comments. One impressive thing you said is that medicine is a religious science. It is how we Hindus consider it as well. The question of payment is very easy. My grandfather was this kind of religious scientist; he would not charge a set fee – just give me what you can. If the patient insisted, he would just make up his mind, depending on his patient's capacity to pay. So, for example, if he is performing the religious ceremony of marriage, he would charge CHF 100 to someone who comes from a poor family and CHF 10,000 for someone who comes from a palace or is rich. So both will know that the charge is according to the ability to pay. He would still treat the patient who could not pay. He would even give the patient money to buy a fruit; this is a part of medicine because he thinks he is doing a good job.

The second comment is about the truth. Don't tell a truth that hurts – that's exactly what is said in Hinduism. Tell the truth, tell them something nice to hear, but truth that hurts the other fellow should not be told.

A. [*Gesundheit*]: Let me share with you: your grandfather has a friend in Talmudic writing. It says that one of the physicians had in his practice a box. After the treatment he would say: if you have money, put it in, if you need money, take some out. The fact that he could continue to work, meaning that people did put something in, says it all. This is a very special attitude: you focus on the wonderful work of the profession and it works.

References

1 Preuss J: Biblisch-talmudische Medizin: Beiträge zur Geschichte der Heilkunde und der Kultur überhaupt. Berlin, Karger, 1911.

2 Habermas, J: On the Pragmatics of Communication; Maeve Cooke, MIT Press, 1998, pp 307–342.

3 Moore AR: Medical humanities: an aid to ethical discussions. J Med Ethics 1977;3:26–32.

4 Moore AR: Sounding board. Medical humanities – a new medical adventure. NEJM 1976;295:1479–1480.

5 Gesundheit B: Die Erlaubnis und Pflicht zu heilen im jüdischen Schrifttum – eine philosophisch-historische Analyse nach Rabbi A.J. Kook (in German). Zeitschrift für Medizinische Ethik 2003; 49:251–261.

6 Oshry E: Responsa from the Holocaust, B. Goldman and Y. Leiman Eds., Judaica Press, 2001.

7 Lichtenstein A: Abortion, a halakhic perspective. Tradition 1991;25:3–12.

8 Pellegrino ED: The metamorphosis of medical ethics. A 30-year retrospective. JAMA 1993;269:1158–1162.

9 Emanuel EJ, Emanuel LL: Four models of the physician-patient relationship. JAMA 1992;267: 2221–2226.

10 Gesundheit B, Hadad E: Maimonides (1138–1204): Rabbi, Physician and Philosopher. Isr Med Assoc J 2005;7:547–553.

Further Reading

– Preuss J: Biblisch-talmudische Medizin: Beiträge zur Geschichte der Heilkunde und der Kultur überhaupt. Berlin, Karger, 1911.

– Jakobovits E: Jewish Medical Ethics – A Comparative and Historical Study of the Jewish Religious Attitude to Medicine and its Practice, 1959.

– Jotkovitz A, Glick S, Gesundheit B: Truth telling in a culturally diverse world. Cancer Invest 2006;24:786–789.

– Steinberg A: Encyclopedia of Jewish Medical Ethics. New York: Feldheim, 2003.

– Encyclopedia of Bioethics: *Information Disclosure. New York: Simon and Schuster, 1995.

– Bleich D: A Physician's Obligation with Regard to Disclosure of Information; in Rosner OF (ed): Medicine and Jewish Law. New York: Yashar Books 1990: 31–63.

Benjamin Gesundheit, MD, PhD
4 Migdal Eder
IL–90433 Alon Shvut (Israel)
E-Mail b.gesund@gmail.com

Religious Perspectives

Pfleiderer G, Battegay M, Lindpaintner K (eds): Knowing One's Medical Fate in Advance. Challenges for Diagnosis and Treatment, Philosophy, Ethics and Religion. Basel, Karger, 2012, pp 87–105

Modern Medicine and My Future Life: A Christian-Theological Perspective

Georg Pfleiderer

Theology Faculty, University of Basel, Basel, Switzerland

Introduction: The Importance of Being Religious

In Western societies, religious belief belongs primarily to the sphere of privacy; it is connected with the idea of individual decisions and convictions which cannot be prescribed to all members of a pluralistic society. Nevertheless, ethical discourses, e.g. on predictive medicine, on questions of the anticipation of individual future can hardly be held without referring to conceptions of good life, of a good future—in the perspective of the respective individual. Such conceptions are always connected with worldviews (*Weltanschauungen*) and their very often religious backgrounds. This is illustrated e.g. in a recent empirical study done in Basel [1] (see also Gabriela Brahier's essay in this volume). Differentiated interviews with pregnant women, having to decide whether to undergo a prenatal genetic test or not, show that in such decisions religious ideas on human life and its meaning are much more involved than it is reflected in most academic debates on such bioethical problems.

There is some discrepancy between the amount of theoretical and practical efforts to improve the communication of medical knowledge and awareness of rather formal questions of ethical autonomy, on the one hand, and the usually reduced intellectual interest on the question: how can a person be helped in his or her attempt to get more clarity on the field of his or basic philosophical and religious convictions? Such partial ignorance of many 'secular' bioethicists regarding this part of ethical decision-making might support consequences that they actually should not, such as irrationalism and the tendencies to obey authoritarian religious authorities.

The following considerations should shed some light on such religious backgrounds. The discussion starts from the standpoint of a modern Christian (namely Protestant) understanding of individual life-conduct, which is based on an general attitude of trust, hope, and responsibility. This Western, modern type of Christian ethics is not categorically hesitant of using instruments of advanced medical techniques.

It argues, however, that the help ethical deliberation and consultancy can give to concerned persons might be limited, as long as they exclude theological reflections on religious horizons and backgrounds in principle.

In order to illustrate some basic ideas of Christian concepts of life, particularly life's end, meaning and afterlife (so-called eschatology), it might be helpful to begin with a sketch of antique belief in fate as a foil of contrast.

Individual Life and Its Future in a Christian Theological Perspective

Anonymous Fate or Destiny by Divine Providence?

The Moirai

In Roman and Greek mythology, there were three goddesses of fate: the so-called Moirai (Latin, *parcae*) or Fates. The first one, Clotho (Nona), spins the fibre of individual destiny, while Lachesis (Decima) interweaves it, and Atropos (Morta) finally cuts it down.

There were different ideas concerning the question whether these deities, and fate in general, were dependent upon the highest God (Zeus, Jupiter), or even the Gods were dependent upon fate. Probably the more archaic Greek idea (Herodot, Homer) was that even the Gods were dependent upon fate, while the later Roman mythology conceived the Parcae as dependent upon Jupiter's will. While this younger concept may reflect influences from monotheistic religions, the older and more archaic Greek imagination, as particularly Homer in the *Iliad* conveys it, even speaks of one goddess, called *moira*. Therefore, one may say that despite their relative plurality and individuality, *moira* basically and originally is an impersonal, anonymous power of fate. Originally, not even the Gods have an influence on fate. Fate is, so-to-speak, 'fatalistic'. Fate is either luck, fortune, fortune or misfortune, bad luck or it is a mixture. Our individual destiny is fate, unchangeably fixed at the moment of our birth.

The Solon Paradox

Ancient Greek philosophy in general is at least latently fatalistic. This is the reason for Solon's famous hesitation to call the most wealthy man on earth, Kroisos, a lucky man. The so-called Solon paradox articulates the dilemma that before the end of our days, we are not able to estimate the quality of our life, but at that end, we do not know it either, because then we are dead. Nevertheless, for Solon himself, the paradox that carries his name, was in fact no paradox: instead of Kroisos, who asked him this question, he named Tellos the most lucky man on earth. Tellos was a more or less ordinary Athenian, who has lived in a flourishing community, has had brave sons, sane grandsons, a good fortune and died an honourable death as a soldier. For Solon, one of the seven wise men of ancient Greece, objective luck and subjective happiness were more or less the same. For modern people, they are different. Luck and fortune are mostly interesting in the first-person perspective: luck is no luck without happiness. Thus, the 'Solon paradox' is a retrospective invention of modernity.

Since the times of Renaissance and Humanism, European intellectuals have sympathized with that ancient concept of anonymous fate. Nevertheless, most of the modern intellectuals did not turn back to the sober fatalism of ancient Greek philosophy which speculated on the question: which was better, to live a more or less happy and lucky life or not having being born at all? Therefore, the burden on subjective fulfilment of life, also the burden which is laid upon us by the uncertainties of our prospective future life, have grown immensely. On this background, the famous end of Albert Camus' existentialist novel [2] is most understood, where Sisyphos should be considered as a happy man.

"Wer immer strebend sich bemüht, den können wir erlösen [3]." Labour and endeavour are the modern solutions of the Solon paradox. The risks and uncertainties of our future life can be overcome by pragmatism. "Hilf Dir selbst, dann hilft Dir Gott" (Help yourself, then God will help you) is the pious version (going even back to the Middle Age), while "Jeder ist seines Glückes Schmied" (Every man is the architect of his own future), is the secular version of such pragmatism, including legitimization and absolution, by procedure.

Providence

It is well known that in Biblical and Christian theology, things are different. Individual fate and individual future life are believed to lie in the hand of God. God, in his divine foreknowledge, knows and foresees our destiny, our deeds and our future; moreover, God is also the latent power behind all earthly action and events. With his almighty providence, he guides and navigates the ships of our lives through the ocean of time— the technical term is *gubernatio* (originally, steering [of a ship]) in classic dogmatics. Nevertheless, such divine providence must not be understood as an absolute determination of life, as it does not prevent the idea of human freedom; on the contrary, it wants to name its transcendental condition, i.e. the absolute subjectivity of God is the *raison d'être* of any finite subjectivity.

Such finite freedom is however limited, not as a consequence of divine determination or anonymous fate, but as a consequence of the wrongful use of freedom, of sin. For every individual this 'fatal' involvement into sin is a fact, it has always already happened. To put in traditional theological ideas: no human being is free like Adam and Eve before the fall. We are, so to speak, all children of Adam and Eve after the fall. Nevertheless, Christians also believe that the consequences of the fall are overcome by the liberation of Jesus Christ. By believing in him, freedom is possible.

Therefore, in Christianity the three *Moirai* are replaced by the triune God. One might say it is God, the creator, who spins our fibre of life, it is Christ, the son, who interweaves our present life with those of others, and it finally is the Holy Spirit in which the future of our life (and within this future, sooner or later, its end) is merged.

Thus, in a Christian understanding of destiny, all fatal associations must be understood as negated and overcome. 'Destiny' is related to 'destination': each individual has a certain aim and perspective in life. He or she is called to find and follow it.

Individual Destiny

Although it was not until the rise of modernity in the 18th century that Christian theologians emphasized the importance of individuality in anthropology, there is a certain inclination towards individualism and appreciation of individual biographical life already at the biblical cradle of Christianity, in the New Testament. A religion whose central theological task is it to relate a certain finite biography of a particular individual (Jesus of Nazareth) to the essence and the being of the absolute, infinite, universal deity is actually compelled to reflect on the meaning of individuality.

The most visible effect of this reflection is the Christian concept of faith—faith is an individual act; in faith, no one is exchangeable by another person, not the wife by the husband, not the children by the parents. In a strict sense of the word, belief is not a social but an individual practice. There are of course groups of believers, there is a church, a community, and there is a common or a shared belief, nevertheless, the act of belief is essentially individual. The objects of vocation in the New Testament, the first disciples, are depicted as particular individuals. Even baptism is individual: "I've called you upon your name, you are mine".

To be sure, belief means the incorporation into a new social body, into the church as the community of believers, which is believed to be the body of Christ. "In Christ, you all are one" (Gal 3,28) —but they do not lose their individuality, they rather gain it—it is the individual charismata which make the church live. Indifference and uniformity are not indices of Christian life and freedom but of sin.

Christian Understanding of Personal Future, Death and Afterlife

Two Formative Tensions

The relationship of the individual to his or her future life is, in Christianity, at least in traditional Western Christianity, determined by strong tensions. They are two-fold and precisely these:

1 The tension between redemption which has already happened (in Jesus Christ) and future redemption (in the 'day of Judgment').

2   The tension between finite, carnal and infinite, transcendent, spiritual life.

These strong and two-fold tensions are formative for Christianity. The events and deeds of my finite future life, how I behave, what I will experience, are equally appreciated and filled with enormous meaning, but also, they are very much relative and relieved of heavy impositions.

During the 2,000 years of Christian history, as well as regarding the variety of respective different groups and churches, this two-fold tension is interpreted in an extreme variety of forms. Let us just pick two important particular movements: The Reformation and Enlightenment.

Reformation Theology: The Prerogative of Justification (Grace)

(1) Reformation theology, in the shape of Martin Luther or John Calvin, very much concentrated on the first part of the first tension, i.e. the work of redemption. Exactly spoken, the work of justification or atonement, is done once, forever and sufficiently in the events of the life, death and resurrection of Jesus Christ. No person on earth is able (nor forced) to add in his or her life something substantial to the meaning and the value of this world-changing chain of events. The future, every future of everyone who believes in Jesus Christ, is bright and open, however dark, sorrowful and viewless his or her empiric life and future actually are.

Like Paul, Luther and even more Calvin hurried to emphasize that this fundamentally good message for the perspective of individual future life must not be taken as a permission to live without ethical efforts and social responsibility; on the contrary, the knowledge of this passed justification is entailed with intrinsic necessity the attendance to live one's life in service for the interests of one's neighbour, that is, to live a life in so-called 'sanctification'.

(2) In addition, both Luther and Calvin also agreed in Paul's claim that by far much better than any future in this finite life would and will be the future life which we may expect after death. The intensity and realism of this belief in the transcendent life (after life) for the Reformed (and not only Reformed) Christianity, until at least early 18th century, is hardly to be overestimated. It was, as it is still well known, much more than a theological doctrine, it was the widely shared assumption and the core of Christianity for more or less all Christians. The music of Johann Sebastian Bach or the hymns of Paul Gerhardt give testimony of this religious reality.

Enlightenment: Spiritualisation of Afterlife Conceptions

It was the movement of *Enlightenment* which changed this scene more or less radically. However, although under the influence of Enlightenment since late 18th century, the average European Christian lost the 'self-evident' concept of a 'realistic' understanding of afterlife. Actually, he or she did not lose any kind of such belief; instead, a great spiritualisation and 'ethicalization' of the concepts of transcendent life took place.

This spiritualisation happened surprisingly enough without a major crisis in the Christian religion. The realistic and colourful images of transcendent life were not replaced in a coup de force by usually abstract ideas, but rather slowly and from generation to generation with more emphasis; it was replaced by a more spiritual and—particularly in the heyday of Enlightenment—a more ethical understanding of its meaning.

Nevertheless, and despite its so-to-speak formal character, this transformation of fundamental religious assumptions did go along with some remarkable changes in their material content. Although the enlightened understanding of transcendence stressed the ethical effects of its meaning, and, in turn, the idea of social justice and of a God who repays and rewards our good deeds, enlightenment-theology particularly and even more philosophy went to great trouble to illustrate the other side of this concept: the rigorous and strict side of God and of ultimate Judgement. The concept of hell and eternal punishment had lost its plausibility and, during the 19th century, all the efforts of conservative pastors to keep it present in the minds of their flock became more and more fruitless. Punishment was also spiritualized and internalized; it was transformed in the concept of a mostly bad—at least in the 19th century, notoriously bad—Christian consciousness.

Thus, within about two centuries the modern individual, the modern Christian individual, was born. What made this birth possible on Christian religious grounds was the fact that it actually was not an entirely new birth but rather a rebirth of an older theological concept. In a way, the realistic, physical, supranatural understanding of an afterlife that dominated the phenomenology of Christian imagery and thinking before modernity, had in fact always been rather a kind of external skin of the core of the religious convictions. Under the surface of its epistemological realism, e.g. Reformation theology, in fact, it had a 'spiritual' understanding of afterlife and transcendence. Likewise, in the New Testament itself, the images of transcendent life, i.e. the concepts of a bodily resurrection, never were communicated with the claim of a literal, 'physical' reality. Otherwise, the fact that the event of the returning of Jesus Christ did actually not happen within one or two generations as the early Christians, even Paul, had expected, would have caused a much deeper crisis in Christianity than it actually had. Therefore, for some 2,000 years, Christian eschatology could mix and combine elements from a mostly Platonic dualism of eternal soul and finite material, flesh on the one side and a rather Biblical understanding of a resurrection of the body on the other side. The story of the bodily ascension of the resurrected Jesus is only told in one of the four gospels, respectively—in the Acts of the Apostles connected to one of the four, the gospel of Luke. The most spiritual gospel, particularly the one of John, could perfectly do without such theological realism.

It continued on, with an at least particular inclination or affinity to an idealistic ontology and anthropology in the sense of Platonic philosophy. This was typical for classical Christian modernity, the period between about 1750 and about 1920. With no doubt, this concept has its problematic aspects. It is often accompanied by a more or less strong tendency to devalue the meaning of the body for the individual person. There is a kind of ascetic somatophobia in many versions of Christian Platonism.

'Holistic Humanity' ('Der Ganze Mensch')

It is then one of the merits of 20th century theology—a theology whose cradle stood, to put it tragically, near the trenches of the first technical war in history i.e. World War I, and not least of the theology of Karl Barth—to uncover this tendency and to lead back to a more biblical understanding of Christian eschatology and anthropology.

In this context and particularly in the light of the unprecedented cruelties (at least concerning their quantity) human beings could infect with their fellow co-creatures and their bodies in the wars and the extermination camps of the last century, Christian theology had to learn a new understanding of pain, illness, but also of positive (full of relish) affections of the body. They are not to overcome with simple appeals to a stronger belief in 'the better and higher part' of human beings or with remarks on the relative meaning and externality of everything which happens to the body—'only' to the body—if only the soul and the spirit would be able to overcome it.

Christianity had to take a new lesson on the understanding of its own Christological roots. Therefore, it developed theological concepts of an 'holistic humanity' ('der ganze Mensch') [4].

For Christian ethics in the tradition of Western 20th century theology, it is now mostly out of the question that the biblical talking of 'eternal life' must be understood as a metaphor for the eternal meaning of this individual finite life here on Earth that ends with physical death. Instead, eternal life is not a second life with a second material or immaterial body, but more the deeper meaning of this life—this finite, individual, biographical, unique life—it is this life but 'viewed with the eyes of God'.

Classical Christian theology assumed that there is an empirical (sensitive and conscious) participation of the individual in this divine view: "we will see his glory and delightfulness"; modern theology takes this 'seeing' as a metaphor for the idea that there is an absolute meaning of every particular finite life, which is only present in the eyes of an absolute observer of this life. Regardless of how participation in this divine observation of our life will be, according to Christian theology, it is this outlook of individual future life that should be the frame of all our dealings with the challenges of prognostic knowledge.

Some Consequences for Christian Bioethics of Individual 'Future Life'

No Affront Against Modern Medical Techniques

From a Christian theological perspective, as I conceive it, there is not only no general verdict against the application and the development of advanced technologies of medical predictive knowledge; on the contrary, there is an ethical duty to develop and apply such advanced technologies in order to help people compassionately against their pains and diseases. Therefore, modern Christian ethics also plead for the use of available modern techniques of medical prognosis. Not to make use of them while they exist and while and as long they could lead to medical treatment of diseases which are curable, would mean a wrongful understanding of the virtue of unconcern.[1]

Against Naturalism

Nevertheless, there is a sense of sobriety in a Christian doctrine of finite life and its eternal meaning which should lead to a reasonable management of such medical instruments and information. Such reasonable use means to calculate the probability but also never to take even percentages of 99.9% as indications for an interpretation of human life as being strictly determined by the power of an anonymous nature and, therefore, a blind fate.

In the meantime, not only for those well-known biological reasons, prognoses on the basis of genetic testing particularly must not be taken as an argument for a naturalistic determination of human life. Moreover, this is wrong for theological reasons. Divine providence, as the foundation of the possibility of human freedom, undermines naturalistic determination as it opens the space for an interpretation of the meaning and the sense of an individual life, which makes it completely independent from the questions of how long and how comfortable it was.

Against Religious-Metaphysical Escapism

Christian interpretations of life inspired by the Bible will disclaim a metaphysical escape against the threat of vanity, occurring on the foundation of a naturalistic perspective on life, by contemplating, e.g. a religious or metaphysical theory of reincarnation. The belief in a series of reincarnations is hard to synthesize with the concept of the central meaning of the uniqueness of the individual finite life which is formative for Christian anthropology. Trouble and anxiety regarding one's personal

---

[1] Unconcern can definitely be a form of confidence and trust. As such, it is highly appreciated. However, it can also be a form or carelessness against oneself and others dependent upon myself.

future is part of the human finite existence. Thus, the Christian concept of the divine providence is very different from a religious-metaphysical doctrine of reincarnation; it stands in opposition to all kinds of naturalism, be they biological or metaphysical.

The Freedom of Hope

Trouble and anxiety can not be overcome solidly by such doctrines of reincarnation. More promising is an attitude that starts with the awareness that all our personal efforts to make our lives meaningful are limited and finally insufficient. A feeling of sense and meaningfulness of a life, which, regarding its biological process, seems to be more or less definitely determined by the foreseeable process of a particular disease. Such a meaningfulness can only be experienced as a gift of an absolute divine subject who—as Immanuel Kant put it, as a philosophical postulate of pure reason—stands at the end of both of causalities: the causality of nature and of that of freedom (compare with Kant in 5). It is this freedom, the freedom of hope, on which the freedom to use medical prognostic tools without becoming reamed in the double bind of anxiety and carelessness, may proceed.

Predictive Medicine: Challenges to a Modern Christian Ethics of Individual Future Life

Classical Medical Prevention: Example of Breast Cancer

Recent studies have questioned the utility of the broad breast cancer prevention programmes as they exist in many European countries. The basic argument is that the actual number of cases of death avoided by these screening programs is very little. The collateral damage of a much higher rate of unnecessary breast surgery, namely breast amputation, would be much higher. This argument of collateral damage is per se cogent. Nevertheless, it raises the normative questions: is such balancing allowed? Particularly, is it allowed to balance death cases with cases of unnecessary medical disfigurement? In the perspective of modern Christian ethics, the answer is no! Life, the existence, of human beings is an absolute value. It must not be the object of a calculating balance. The only exemption of this rule is the conflict of life against life. The solution to the problem can only be a practical one: efforts must be taken to reduce the number of such unnecessary cases of 'collateral damage'. It is a question of quality control and quality management in the health system.

End-of-Life Decisions

End-of-life decisions are usually based on some kind of predictive medicine, at the very least, on a medical prognosis of the future process of the respective illness. The particularity of those decisions depends on the terminal nature of the disease. This implies that usually it is impossible to find out whether an alternative decision would have been the better solution. It is a 'Solonic' disclosure paradox.

Is there a general option for modern Christian ethics to avoid such situations? I believe there is not, at least not for the modern Christian ethics as it is conceived here. This answer is based on the assumption that there are medically influenced situations in which a decision about the continuation of life is unavoidable.

The Concept of 'Rational Suicide' ('Bilanzsuizid')

In the perspective of modern Christian ethics, it is ethically problematic to use a concept of a rationally calculated suicide, that is, a suicide based on the idea of a soberly formulated 'balance sheet' of one's own life and its further perspective. The concept of such a so-called 'rational suicide' steps out of the Solon-paradox, it negates the principle openness and 'unknownness' of our future life. In addition, the concept is usually based on a strong idea of individual autonomy, which assumes that the perspectives of others who might be interested in the continuation of my life are, at first, of lower importance than my own perspective, and, at second, I do not have to ask such (potential) others for their interests but can imagine them myself.

The concept of 'rational suicide' is the most radical, the most practical, and the most common concept of negating the questions which are posed by the openness and 'unknownness' of our future life. If it is the basic idea of Christian ethics to keep this horizon open, then for principal reasons the concept of 'rational suicide' is not applicable in this context.

Saying this does, nevertheless, not mean to claim: there are no true end-of-life decisions at all in the perspective of such a theological ethics. To be sure, there are such decisions; there is no duty to prolong life with all means of modern medicine. Human life can reach a kind of fulfilment, of conclusion, of roundness, but perhaps also of pain and depletion that it would make no sense to prolong it with the use of technical instruments. Nevertheless, this estimation must, in principle, be tied strictly to the first-person perspective. If a person is unable to perform his or her will, ways must be found to find it out. A living will which is formulated precisely and contemporarily gives the best and obligatory hints to that will.

Regarding Death: Fulfilment, Fragmentariness and Openness

In the Bible, the patriarchs died—as the formula puts it, "in a good old age. . . and full of years" or "full of days" (Abraham, Gen 25,8; Isaac, Gen 35,29). Max Weber [6] stated that such fulfilment would not be available any more under the conditions of modernity. This thinking is typical for the spirit of modernity we all participate in and it is particularly quite close to that of the emphatic campaigners of life prolongation today. It is, however, not completely convincing. A complete negation of any kind of fulfilment in life, would mean to negate the possibility of individual experience of sense and meaning. Individual life, in general and particularly in modernity, is always fragmentary. As in the fragments of sculptures there can be, nevertheless, hints to a totality and unity, even in their fragmented nature. An anticipation of totality and roundness in life can be imagined that is not subject to knowledge—not to medical knowledge—but to belief and hope.

Genetic Testing as a Litmus Test for Christian Ethics of Individual Future Life

The Mythology of Genetic Testing

Dealing with genetic testing is something like a litmus test in the Christian ethics of the individual future life. Genes are, so to speak, the *Moirai* (goddesses of fate) in modernity: they seem to determine our fate in an absolute and also somehow anonymous way. It is curious that in both semantics or 'mythologies' the symbol of the *fibre*, the string, plays such an important role: the fibre of our fate is the DNA-string. The determination of our future lies in the past of evolution. Like in ancient tragedies, family ties often beyond our knowledge and active memory are crucial for our destiny. Like the silk-string which holds the sword of Damocles, curses inscribed in our genes seem to hang over us.

Genetic testing and genetic engineering are the techniques which carry the hope of an unveiling of such archaic curses placed on humanity, an opportunity to influence our destiny and to get rid of those dark shadows covering our future. Particularly in the early days of genetic research, the hopes pinned on these techniques were similar to that of those archaic cultures that pinned on a mighty blessing that would ban the curses of fate.

Such quasi-religious desires tied to these new medical techniques have mostly disappeared and, particularly in Europe, they were often replaced by the opposite; a new and even worse fatalism was introduced. For many people, the foreseeable availability of cheap genetic-test kits, which would give almost everyone the chance to foresee his or her personal future—to learn about the probability of major genetic diseases, the consequences for life insurance, for long-dated contracts of employments, but also maybe for the decision to marry certain persons, to have children with her or him, etc.—are rather a nightmare and actually a new curse on the future of public and personal life.

Meanwhile, we have learned that the prognostic exactness or accuracy of these genetic tests is, in general, much lower than originally expected. Genes are not the compelling schedule, the definite 'blueprint' of our biological future life. Most of the diseases which have a genetic condition are not mono- but multi-genetically conditioned. For many diseases, this implies that a genetic test indicates only a more or less rough probability than to the actuality of developing a certain disease. Furthermore, these genetic-test kits have increased the problem of translating the rather abstract probability values into personal life plans. Clearly, there are monogenetic diseases with a very high predictability, like Huntington's chorea or cystic fibrosis, but even concerning multi-genetic diseases, the psychological, judicial and ethical problems caused by such genetic tests are still serious enough.

A Christian Attitude towards Genetic Testing

Is there a general ethical perspective concerning genetic testing on the ground of such a modern Christian ethics of personal life conduct as it is outlined here? I believe there is. To put in the form of a thesis: the string of our life is not a string, woven or cut by an anonymous power, be it a goddess or nature, but it is the string of the story of our personal life. The basic conviction of Christian belief is that there is no situation in life and no future perspective that is so desolate that a meaningful life conduct is in principle not possible any more. Even if we knew the exact minute and the precise condition of our death, or the moment of a disease outbreak, the freedom to live a life worthy to live until this moment with an open horizon would not be destroyed.

To be clear, this does not mean that genetic testing is a harmless affair in the perspective of such an ethics. There are still plenty of psychosocial, political and judicial problems to be solved. Probably the most striking psychosocial problem is the making of the so-called 'pre-symptomatic person'. It is a kind of stigmatisation, a social exclusion, or an ostracism, which bans a person from the realm of the 'normal' people years before the respective person becomes ill. Christian ethics oppose both the social exclusion and, even more so, the exclusion executed in advance.

In general, the right not to know is crucial here; no one must be forced to learn more on his or her genetic structure than he or she wants to learn. The responsible freedom Christian ethics plead for concerning my own life conduct and my future life, does not contain an imperative to collect all available information on my personal life or on the lives of those I am living closely with, i.e. my wife, my children and so on, rather, in the contrary. In the Bible, and not by accident, fortune telling is very different from legitimate prophecy. The first is connected with superstition, the latter with true belief. True Prophecy is always the announcement of the superiority of God even over a seemingly hopeless prognosis. There is on the other side no complete ban on such knowledge. Insofar as it helps to live a responsible life, which is very different from a life operated by the desire of total self-control; it can be helpful and even demanding in certain situations. Christian life stories can never be tragedies.

Genetic Diseases and the Threat to Lose Identity

In a sensitive study, Monica Konrad [7] showed distinctly how complex and how demanding the decision to make a genetic test can be for members of families in which Huntington's disease has appeared. Some of the persons she has interviewed carried that decision about them for a long time, in one case even for several years. As Huntington's chorea is a strongly hereditary disease, with a 50% probability of an offspring of a ill parent to receive the disease, a special problem with it is the disclosure dilemma, particularly concerning adolescent children. Another major problem is the effect of positive, but also negative diagnoses, can have on family ties. The diagnosis tends to split the family: one part which is pre-symptomatic or symptomatic ill and another part which is not. Another major problem is caused by the frequent fact that members of such families very often have terrifying experiences with this disease during their childhood when a close member of the family, e.g. the mother or father, had been ill. Commonly, such an experience was traumatic for the then children.

Monica Konrad's study showed how different are the individual ways of dealing with such a situation and with the question whether and when to make a genetic test. It also shows that for the persons concerned, it might be the most difficult task not to lose their self-control or at least to keep up the impression as if they had not lost it. This is related to the extreme challenges that such a scenario or the risk to get Huntington's disease has for those persons. The study also showed that the probably most striking anxiety was caused by the threat to lose self-control, in connection with a lost of his or her identity by a severe change of character. This is probably similar to the threat of getting Alzheimer's disease (although only very few of all Alzheimer's cases are genetically caused) and therefore can potentially be diagnosed by a genetic test.

With no doubt, Alzheimer's and Huntington's disease belong to the most dreadful and challenging attacks on a person's integrity. This could exactly be the reason why in modern societies it is so difficult to handle them and particularly to deal with the certainties and uncertainties of the respective predictive medicine.

Personal integrity and self-control are essential for our self-image and for our estimation of what a good life should be. With medical enlightenment, so to speak, our cultural patterns to deal with mental diseases were changed—mostly for the better, but also for the worse—for the persons concerned.

We usually do not call somebody who has a dementia a lunatic or a madman any more; modern societies have lost the idea that such persons were obsessed by demons that must be exorcised. Modern societies have, however, also lost the idea that such a person is torched by a demon and must be helped, or that he or she in a mental state that is closer to the divine sphere and therefore should be treated with particular respect. In addition, modernity has emphasized the importance of rational self-control and of a stable identity, calculable for others to such an extent that it actually tends to exclude a person who is beyond these requirements from social estimation. Medical enlightenment and common moral values seem to be more tolerant in these questions; even so, it might be that there is a lot of political correctness in play. Otherwise, it would hardly be understandable that, in the first-person perspective, the fear of getting a mental disease is so extreme in modern societies. We are trained, at least in theory, to tolerate any person on Earth affected with a mental disease, or the threat of it, but not in ourselves.

It is, to my eyes, an important task for Christian ethics as well as in society in the intercourse with persons concerned to counteract these problematic tendencies of modernity. Such a counteraction could be the opportunity a disease like Alzheimer's provides for the society. It could help us to change the normative image of the self-controlled identical person. Indeed, the concept of a stable identity is mostly a thin lacquer and autobiographical authenticity is always accompanied by orchestration. The self is rather naturally fragmented than it is identical with itself, and identity is not such much an achievement of the individual but an ascription by others or mainly by the self—as an other. In addition to such insights, Christian ethics would insist on the idea that it is not one of the fatal anonymous modern goddesses or *moirai,* so-called society, evolution or nature, but an absolute subject called God who is accessible only by the means of a mostly fragmentary individual who is the subject of that law—and this is the reason why people may believe that the strings of their fragmentary life are knotted beyond their backs to a net that will hold them when they fear to sink.

Predicting My Offspring: Is There a Christian Eugenics?

Parenthood must be accompanied by responsibility. There are the rights of the unborn (H. Jonas) to us, at least of those unborn who will be born by our coop-eration. Responsibility is, as Max Weber put it rightly, always responsibility for the future. Therefore, responsibility must be accompanied by the readiness to collect a reasonable amount of knowledge about the respective future, e.g. of a pregnancy, a birth and the child which is on the way into this life. This is—for the Christian ethics as conceived here—the ethical *raison d'être* for prenatal diagnosis, at least concerning diseases or disabilities that can be medicated or treated. Yet, most of the ethical prob-lems discussed in the realm of pre-implantation and prenatal diagnosis start beyond this line; they have to do with some sort of eugenics.

Is there a general verdict against eugenics on the ground of modern Christian eth-ics? Yes, there is. As many contemporary philosophers, e.g. Jürgen Habermas [8], have showed, individual freedom presupposes the idea of an anonymous and con-tingent nature as donator of our individual shape and not the particular interests of one or two individuals or, even worse, groups or societies. Nevertheless, as Habermas states with Hannah Arendt, the philosophical hints to nature as the reference and the condition for an "indisposable beginning"[2] beyond all human history seems to

---

[2] "unverfügbarer Anfang", see 8, p 101.

be problematic. In this age of genetic information, such a nature beyond any human disposition turns out to be a fiction. In this historical moment, nature has lost its transcendental function for the self-identification of free human subjects. The second candidate of such a reference, which "detracts individual freedom from the availability of other persons"[3] according to Habermas himself, is God. Nevertheless, Habermas does not discuss this 'candidate' for an absolute point of reference of individual self-development, whereas modern Christian ethics suggest to do so.

On theological grounds, there is a general, but not a total verdict against eugenics, based on a prenatal, or even pre-implantation, genetic testing. It is not completely forbidden to discuss whether there might be exemptions from the general rule, not to influence the genetic shape of my offspring. God might be more tolerant than Habermas. There might be certain situations, e.g. families affected by Huntington's disease, in which an evaluation of the higher right is tolerable. Of course, there is—as particularly Roman-Catholic moral theologians argue at this point—no right of a sane offspring. Nevertheless, a categorical insistence on the potential personality of each human embryo also leads into logical and moral contradictions. Threatening diseases like Huntington's chorea are candidates for decisions with pre-implantation genetic diagnosis, and which should probably be left to those who have to live with it.

Questions and Answers

Q. [*Battegay*]: I was wondering if you could, and perhaps also Benjamin Gesundheit, comment on the differential stance that the Judeo-Christian world—if we can put it under one roof—takes in particular on your last point on pre-implantation testing and pre-implantation consultation. It is commonplace in the Jewish religion to advise couples, actually, prior to getting married, about the risk of a heritable disease. What is the position of the Christian faith on that?

A. [*Pfleiderer*]: There is actually not only one Christian position on PID but many of them. The differences mostly depend upon different concepts of prenatal human life. For most Roman Catholic ethicists prenatal life is in general and from the moment of insemination the life of an in principle complete individual human being. Therefore, embryo selecting is considered as unmoral as abortion. In Protestant ethics there are different positions. Some agree with Roman Catholics in this bio-ontological perspective, but there are also more liberal positions which point to the importance of social relationships as a necessary condition for the development of individual life. Regarding PID, representatives of the latter position also often plead for an ethics of responsibility which points to the fact that a prohibition of PID usually leads to an increase of the abortion rate. Despite this emphasis of the importance of social relations this position does not devaluate the ethical meaning of individuality,

---

[3] "der Verfügbarkeit anderer Personen entzieht", ibid.

on the contrary, it is referring to a biographical model of individuality which is different from an understanding of human life conducted by the value of the life of the family or the tribe as a whole. Such religious views can be found in traditional Islam, in several Asian Religions, but also in Orthodox Judaism.

[*Gesundheit*]: I agree that there might be a difference in the status of the family. I think a very important issue for prenatal testing is that according to Jewish law, compared to the Protestant methodical approach, there is the possibility for abortion. It is not strictly forbidden like in the Catholic approach. Having said that, it makes it possible for the mother if she wants it, for example for Tay-Sachs disease, a classical Jewish genetic disease. In the beginning, it was not clear if the diagnosis was accurate or not. Once that was done, it was certainly allowed. The Rabbinical authorities have clearly said the earlier the better–there are discussions about that. People who were familiar with the medical aspects certainly supported it because it entails terrible suffering for the child and the family. It is the status of the abortion, which makes the difference. Especially in a situation when you can predict the future and you can do something about it.

Q. [*Pfleiderer*]: In my eyes, there is a problem here: How do we deal today with historic religious perspectives on bioethical problems? A religious thinker of the 3rd century argues on the basis of a medical knowledge and view of the early phases of human life which is completely different from ours.

A. [*Gesundheit*]: First of all, it is interesting to see how this source which I presented is interpreted, and the very interesting theories in the texts and the traditions. But what I found in the Responsa, meaning the Rabbinical answers to these questions, was particularly interesting, not only what is said in the sources, but also what is their rationale. Other approaches said: if you go through all the tests which can be done–the person gets crazy. Here is a very important consideration–what is important might not be source related. What is good for the patient? If all the tests which could be done and all the possible investigations which can be found on the Internet were to be carried out and believed, each pregnancy would become a terrible stress. Some Rabbis argued: do the most important ones and others, you have to trust in God. Of course, you have to trust in God. For the balance between these issues, and this might be a general comment, too much knowledge might very often be very stressful for the family, with all the Jewish grandmothers involved and everybody giving their good ideas and advice. The whole pregnancy becomes very stressful.

[*Pfleiderer*]: Exactly, but this indicates that not only our medical knowledge has changed since the ancient world but also our understanding of society and social life. We do not live in a patriarchal society any more, women – pregnant women for instance – are considered as autonomous human beings and their behavior is not dependent on the permission of their husbands.

Q. [*Mr. Gyr*]: I was fascinated by the difference between soul and life. As far as I know, Christianity has come through such hues too? In the Middle Ages, there was this discussion: when does life begin? If they had the question [then] of prenatal diagnostics, they wouldn't have had a problem now. So then, it is a new view for Christianity right now. What do you think about it? It actually has changed to more a rigid view. At that time [Middle Ages], it was considered that the soul started at six weeks or more after conception. When did they believe life started or when soul started?

A. [*Pfleiderer*]: Thomas Aquinas thought that the unification of body and soul does not happen at the moment of insemination but later: boy souls would come into the body at the 40th day after conception, while for girl souls it would take around another 40 days longer. Even such ideas were gender-coded, as you see. Therefore, abortions in the very early stages of pregnancy were morally much less problematic as they since became in modern Catholicism.

Q. [*Battegay*]: One of the concepts I remember from the last symposium is that Judaism considers creation as incomplete and imperfect, whereas Christianity considers life as perfect at birth? So in Judaism it is not only permissible, it is almost a duty to continue to enhance humanity; so, there is this much more liberal attitude to using this advanced knowledge, such as in this example of pre-implantation diagnosis.

[*Pfleiderer*]: Well, in traditional Christian dogmas a concept of "creation continua" can be found as well – a concept of an ongoing creation which basically means that God is permanently acting in all events and acts of his creatures. In the age of enlightenment such theological concepts could be transformed into ideas of a future moral perfection of man – both in an individual and in a collective sense. Nevertheless, in the 19th and even more the 20th century, Western theology particularly in Europe became very critical of such an optimism of progress, especially regarding ideas of a technical self-perfection of man. Therefore, theology, at least European Christian theology, today is mostly critical towards concepts of human enhancement.

[*Gesundheit*]: I think that the questions of medical ethics are bringing the Jewish sources to a revival. The Rabbi can study it for a lifetime. Asking him these questions makes him aware of what he has to see there. There are very interesting insights, which only science can reveal. I fully agree with you, there is a lot of openness, we are like twins of God. This is a very strong statement—we are full partners. One source was brought to a judge: Truth is a friend of God, this obligation to make advances and progress puts us in a very proactive situation. Having said that, I also agree with you that looking in Israel, for instance, for an answer to the question of the moment of death. For a long time, it was defined by breathing. But the Harvard criteria, which are very practical for heart transplantation, says it will never work if you define death by breathing, there will be no heart transplantation. Therefore, the discussion here–a political discussion with a lot of very interesting agendas, which very often has nothing to do with the sources–but the society creates and shapes new approaches based on the old sources and it is a very interesting process.

Q. [*Regine Kollek*]: I would like to come back to the question of the import of modern science into theology. If you look to pregnancy and abortion, you really have to have the historical perspective. Around the 18th century or so, before we were really able to detect the fetus pregnancy was not known until around the third month.

There were disturbances of the female menses, but in general, there were no abortions because pregnancy more or less could not be detected. There is a very nice work by Barbara Gouden, for example. The impact of modern science now has moralized the human embryo, and I wonder why this didn't happen in Judaism? Because you still have this concept of 'ensoulment'? From my discussion with Islamic scholars, the ensoulment begins after several weeks? So the question is: how do we deal with this relation between modern science and scientific knowledge and religious conception? It seems to be different among different religions–this is one point. The other point is that we look especially at the cases of prenatal diagnosis, the concept of family, or at the social ethics perspective, that is questions like eugenics and selection of embryos. Because, I still think there is a difference between abortion, which is the termination of one pregnancy, and pre-implantation genetic diagnosis, which is selection of one specific embryo among others.

[*Battegay*]: One additional comment as part of the final round. You obviously do not assume that 'modernness' is good. I would challenge that very much. Because we then may have the philosophy and culture that less people will have children, the social framework will fall totally apart, and nature will be really brutalized. Therefore, how good is modern life? I think, because I am also Jewish, I would also like a little bit to challenge the view of modernity. But I think you are very right, modern technical possibilities have brought up new aspects, but that is not the Jewish question about abortion. The question of Judaism is to have one value [the unborn has the highest value] that has value in relation to another value. These are questions that come up whether you like it or not. So, sometimes I think that there is a choice to be made between the mother and the baby. Already, two or three thousand years ago, the mother felt the baby. So I think technically there is a difference, but not in the feelings of the mother. After 8 weeks, as nowadays, the mother felt that she was pregnant, she was vomiting, she felt, she knew that there was a baby. So I would like to challenge that view. Certainly, Christianity as well as Islam have major challenges with modernity. I challenge that modernity is a good thing. It is a fact we have to live with, that's the problem of today, and I would like to throw that back into this very stimulating discussion.

A. [*Pfleiderer*]: I agree: Modernity is a fact that we have to live with, also as religious people. Although it is definitely difficult to talk about something like the ethical value of modernity in general, I would not hesitate to say that modernity contains many positive elements of challenge for religion. It also contains chances for religions to humanize their moral convictions and judgements, particularly in the field of ethics of life.

Q. [*Klaus Lindpaintner*]: I just want to slip in a cautious defence of modernity, in a very limited sense. Some of the theories underlying religious and ethical doctrines are just rejected by modern science. For example, the theory of successive ensoulment, which goes back to Aristotle. It is the basis of traditional views, for example, in Muslim countries about the legitimacy or illegitimacy of abortion. The Catholic view, since 1870, is much more modern, saying that life begins with the embryo. This is, in fact, something that has to be and can be accounted as a harmonization with modern science. Of course, this leaves open a huge range of options. However, you yourself rejected the traditional concepts of afterlife, reincarnation and so on, because of this modernization, our concept of man. This does not clarify ethics and doesn't prejudge what the values are. There is a second step—ethics, which I think is a pragmatic undertaking. It is an undertaking which tries to influence discussions and discourses. As William James said, there are some options that are live and some that are dead. So as I understand, within modernization, there are some live options which are controversial and open, and we should concentrate on the live and not on the dead ones. It doesn't mean that modernity is a value in itself, certainly not, but there is a restriction on the avenues we can take.

A. [*Pfleiderer*]: On the one hand, I agree with you: concerning empirical knowledge in the natural sciences we may say that there are hypotheses which are simply outdated. Regarding the humanities and theology on the other hand, in my eyes it is more complicated. Even the Aristotelian concept of an evolutionary ensoulment of the embryo might still have a kind of truth – if you do not take it as an attempt at scientific explanation but as a philosophical interpretation. It then fits quite well into modern concepts of a piecemeal biographical development of individual life which is always a process and the result of a process of contingent interaction with social environment and not only the automatic unfolding of a genetic program.

References

1 Brahier G: Medizinische Prognosen im Horizont eigener Lebensführung. Zur Struktur ethischer Entscheidungsfindungsprozesse am Beispiel der pränatalen genetischen Diagnostik. Tübingen, Mohr Siebeck, 2011 (in press).

2 Albert Camus: Der Mythos des Sisyphos. Deutsch und mit einem Nachwort von Vincent von Wroblewsky, ed 4. Hamburg, Rowohlt Taschenbuch Verlag, 2000, p 160.

3 Johann Wolfgang von Goethe: Faust. Der Tragödie zweiter Teil in fünf Akten. Goethes Werke, Bd III. Textkritisch durchgesehen und mit Anmerkungen versehen von Erich Trunz. Hamburg, Christian Wegner Verlag, 1949, 146–364, p 359 (11936f).

4 Rössler D: Der "ganze Mensch". Das Menschenbild der neueren Seelsorge- lehre und des modernen medizinischen Denkens, im Zusammenhang der allgemeinen Anthropologie. Göttingen, Vandenhoeck und Ruprecht, 1962.

5 Vorländer K (ed): Immanuel Kant: Kritik der praktischen Vernunft, ed 9. Hamburg, Felix Meiner, 1967, pp 142–144 [223–226].

6 Weber M: Wissenschaft als Beruf; in Mommsen WJ, Schluchter W (eds): Wissenschaft als Beruf (1917/19), Politik als Beruf (1919). Tübingen, 1992, 87f.

7 Konrad M: Predictive genetic testing and the making of the pre-symptomatic person: prognostic moralities amongst Huntington's-affected families. Anthropology & Medicine 2003;10:23–49.

8 Habermas J: Die Zukunft der menschlichen Natur. Auf dem Weg zu einer liberalen Eugenik? Frankfurt am Main, Suhrkamp Verlag, 2001.

Prof. Dr. Georg Pfleiderer
Faculty of Theology
University of Basel
Missionsstr. 17a
CH–4055 Basel (Switzerland)
Tel. +41 61 263 78 20, E-Mail georg.pfleiderer@unibas.ch

Pfleiderer G, Battegay M, Lindpaintner K (eds): Knowing One's Medical Fate in Advance. Challenges for Diagnosis and Treatment, Philosophy, Ethics and Religion. Basel, Karger, 2012, pp 106–119

Karma, Contingency, and the 'Point of No Return': Predictive Medicine and Buddhist Perspectives

Jens Schlieter

University of Bern, Bern, Switzerland

> We do not know what will come first—
> The next day or the next life
> (Tibetan saying)

Knowing One's Medical Fate in Asia?

What does it mean to know one's medical fate in advance? How do adherents of non-European religious traditions in Asia conceptualize prospective health conditions? How do they evaluate new techniques of prediction in regard to various forms of genetic testing at the beginnings of life (see 1), on the one hand, or, on the other hand, prognostic prediction in the midst of a person's life or the imminent fate at its end? Do they stick to explanations of fate and contingency that might differ only slightly from those convictions we are used to perceive as more or less generally shared? Or do adherents of Asian traditions such as Buddhist, Hindu, or Ruist/Confucianist traditions conceptualize 'fate', 'future', 'genetics', and 'predictions' in a distinctively different manner? Complex and transdisciplinary by nature, these questions have attracted only limited interest by scholars of religion and ethics working with a comparative perspective (see 2). Nevertheless, one should mention the rapidly growing bioethical discourse in Asian traditions, mirrored by the growing body of scientific work on certain 'Asian' ethical attitudes and moral guidelines regarding biomedical practices. In a recent volume on predictive medicine in Asia, Margret Sleeboom-Faulkner states that "accompanying the globalisation of advanced biomedical research, bioethical discussions on the interaction between biotechnology and the community have proliferated over the last four decades, also in Asia" [1, p 11]. Current debates in Asian bioethics seem, at least partially, to be grounded in specific religious views of Asian traditions. Yet, one has to admit that 'religion' does not often rank among the factors accounted for in research on attitudes toward predictive medicine in Asia. According to Sleeboom-Faulkner, recent contributions focus on the question: "To what extent is choice regarding predictive genetic testing in Asia shaped by financial, legal, cultural, social and political factors?" [1, p 19].

Some of the more 'cultural' and 'religious' topics were negotiated in the 'Asian values' debate: adherents of Asian bioethics characterized their approaches (sometimes, politically endowed with post-colonial self-confidence and in strong opposition to 'individualistic Western bioethics') as 'family-centred' ethics, building on the 'laws of nature' and 'weak persons', or as 'relational ethics' of 'shared decision making' [3]. In the case of Buddhist ethics, this approach has been codified e.g. in the Declaration of Interdependence [4]. Quite recently, Buddhist scholars of biomedicine and of Buddhist ethics (e.g. to name a few proponents of the various traditions: Pinit Ratanakul, Shoyo Taniguchi, Karma Lekshe Tsomo, or Soraj Hongladarom) have shown the relevance of these debates for ethical thoughts and decision making from a Buddhist perspective. However, bioethical specialists of various traditions—Christian, Jewish, Muslim, Confucian, Hindu, or Buddhist—show significant differences with regard to which biomedical practices they criticize or refute and to which they allow as neutral or even as desirable form of action (e.g. stem cell research, assisted reproductive technologies and pre-implantation genetic diagnosis, brain death diagnostics and organ donation, etc.). A common first-sight expectation seems to be that religious scholars tend to hold restrictive positions towards new biomedical practices such as genetic diagnostics (and the predictions based on these). Only later, more liberal attitudes of physicians or lay people (the 'secularizing power' of biomedical explanations and institutionalized health practices) force them to abandon their strict positions. Even though this expectation seems plausible, it only describes one special case from a large variety of possible 'religious' attitudes toward biomedical practices. Sometimes, religious specialists emphatically justify certain biomedical practices as favourable, e.g. organ donation as an act of caritas or artificial insemination and prenatal diagnosis as invaluable help for procreation, thereby fulfilling a religious demand, etc.

In this short contribution, however, I am only able to present some preliminary thoughts regarding Buddhist perspectives on predictive medicine. Firstly, I outline the so-called 'point of no return' as a possible hermeneutic tool for serious cases of medical predictions. Secondly, I then turn to the general role of religious notions concerning predictions of health and healing. Thirdly, I portray descriptions of 'medical futility' according to an important medieval source book of Tibetan medicine in order to exemplify the meaning of religion regarding medical prospects of one's future. And finally, I point to bioethical claims of adherents of current Asian Buddhist traditions in which one may find a different normative attitude towards 'predictions' of a patient's— or a non-medicalized, i.e. a 'healthy' person's—health. Even though 'Buddhist', these examples belong to very different historical, cultural, and religious strands. To draw a general conclusion, therefore, is highly problematic if not impossible. Therefore, this contribution can only offer a scant impression of Asian attitudes towards predictive medicine from certain 'islands' in the vast ocean of Asian traditions.

The 'Point of No Return': Its Relevance for Predictive Medicine

I begin with some thoughts on the so-called 'point of no return'. In the early days of propeller-driven aircrafts, the expression 'point of no return' was established to denote a particular moment of a flight. At this important point, captains and navigators were aware of the fact that it was still possible to return to the airport where they had begun the journey with the given amount of fuel. If they decided to cross this 'point of no return', they had to look for a different destination, i.e. another airport, to land. Thus, to reach such a point implies an irrevocable decision: either to turn back or to go on. Opting for the latter, one had to be aware of the risk that unforeseeable conditions might turn the remaining half of the flight and the landing somewhere else into a more risky undertaking—compared to a simple return on the same way. This 'point of no return' can be reached in other circumstances as well, such as an ocean passage or crossing a desert. Quite often, it was—and is—an instant of existential choice and reflection. Whoever is aware of the fact that he is exactly in the middle of a certain passage might be forced to represent this in terms of a crisis, since both his options—to return or to go on—imply a high risk: in terms of travel time and distance, both arrival points are equally far away. One may be tempted to argue that this point is (as self-representation) at work in people who suffer from a 'midlife crisis'— the feeling of being in the midst of one's own life, but may in the best case only have a second half (the poorer, declining half of life, many may add). The assumption of the meaningfulness of such a 'point of no return' can be useful, I would like to argue, for some questions of predictive medicine in general, and for Asian medical traditions in particular.[1]

One of the most prominent and pertinent problems of 'knowing one's medical fate' seems to originate in the situation of being confronted with a diagnosis of an incurable chronic disease, which quite often implies the prediction of a limited lifespan. In this situation, the 'point of no return' (a) may be combined with the termination of causal therapy, and a shift to palliative care. Another 'point of no return' (b) could be seen in 'persistent vegetative states' or comatose patients affected by an irreversible brain stem dysfunction (an indicator of death in various countries).

For the 'subjective' or first-person perspective, for the one who receives such a fatal diagnosis, the 'point of no return (a)' will, however, differ from the third-person perspectives implied in the 'point of no return (b)'. When they receive such a diagnosis in the pre-final phase, many patients may be over-optimistic and hope for some

---

[1] To state a 'point of no return' does not imply the appraisal of a general 'human finitude'—the latter may, due to its roots in Christian theology (see 5, 6), be problematic if transferred to non-theistic traditions (e.g. as an equivalent of 'impermanence' in Buddhism).

spontaneous healing; or they count on the possibility of an inaccurate diagnosis. For the physicians and other observers from an external, third-person perspective the 'point of no return' should be assessed and substantiated according to the actuarial—the statistical—data available. Beyond a doubt, empathizing family members or other close people to the patient will, nevertheless, try to 'adopt' the first-person perspective. To them, the classical bioethical dilemma consists in the problem whether or not prognostic information should be made explicit to patients. It seems, as some studies have revealed, that attitudes of Japanese physicians towards the 'disclosure' of a progressive cancer diagnosis differ considerably from middle European norms (see 7 and footnote).[2]

In general, the complex "art of predictive medicine" has to deal with the first/third-person-gap and conjectures regarding the patient's reaction—in the words of Monica Konrad:

> "Whatever the specific test outcome, enhancing predictability in human genomics produces the inescapable irony one may never know in advance quite how any given testee will respond. The art of predictive medicine is characterised by the richness of contingency and conjecture that is the human condition" [8, p 146].

How the 'point of no return (b)', reached in the process of dying, will be experienced from a first-person perspective is something that we may never 'know'—possibly it is something not to be 'known' at all, if we follow the line of thought of the sociologist Niklas Luhmann [9] (translated by myself):

> "One's own death may be represented as the end of life, but not as the end of consciousness. [. . .] Consciousness cannot come to an end; it just disappears. [. . .] Therefore, consciousness is not able to know itself as something that can be brought to an end, and, due to this fact, it assigns to itself [. . .] eternal life, just by refraining to consider all known contents [of consciousness]."

This description may lead one to acknowledge the strong impact of cultural as well as religious attitudes on the perception of the 'point of no return' and its effect on 'consciousness' or the 'eternal soul'. Explaining attitudes of the Confucian traditions, Edwin Hui points to these "non-scientific factors" in the perception of "futility":

> "A futile medical procedure has been defined as one that cannot achieve its stated goals or produce its expected benefits with an acceptable level of probability regardless of repetition and duration of treatment [. . .] But in practice, because goals and benefits as well as estimations of probability are dependent on both scientific and non-scientific factors that may affect perceptions of the illness and the predictions of outcome, the notion of futility is a highly value-laden and culturally-bound issue. For this reason, to date no objective unambiguous criteria have emerged in the determination of the futility of any medical treatment, and most writers agree that value choices are involved in most futility judgments" [10, p 128].

---

[2] "In Japan, historically, physicians have withheld discussing cancer diagnoses directly with patients. However, since the early 1990s, due to the increased understanding and adoption of informed consent policy and practice, physicians have gradually begun to inform patients of their cancer diagnosis in clinical practice. In many cases, however, details regarding prognosis are still concealed from patients, especially if the condition is incurable" [7].

We may summarize that the first- and the third-person perspective in regard to the 'knowledge' of one's medical fate may differ substantially vis-à-vis most serious, life-threatening circumstances, and, moreover, that these perspectives may encompass much more than the scientifically based medical knowledge.

Contingency and Karma—or Why Religious Specialists Compete with Medical Specialists in Forecasting 'Medical Fate'

I now broaden the view and present some thoughts on the specific functions of religious interpretations of human life. According to philosophers and sociologists such as Luhmann or Hermann Lübbe, the specific function of religious interpretation is to cope with contingency. 'Contingency' in a more narrow sense can be defined as a state of affairs that could have been other than it is—in contrast to a state of affairs that is necessary because there is no possible alternative to it. In relation to statements: all propositions are contingent that are true in some cases and false in others.

Although Aristotle had already defined 'contingency', one may argue that the existential outlook of 'contingency' is deeply intertwined with the history of Christian thought. In monotheistic traditions, the formula of the strategy for coping with contingency should, according to Luhmann, in some way or the other be connected with God. From the first-person perspective of a religious person, the answer to the question why he or she is affected by a certain disease may build on an interpretation such as 'this happens according to the will of God', or, that it does not affect the eternal life of the soul, etc.

However, radical contingency is not only a dominant strand of certain Protestant Christian traditions, it pertains to secular worldviews, too.[3] Granted that religions contribute to coping with contingency, one may surmise that different (normative) coping strategies might exist in different religions. Since Buddhist normative sources share the opinion of an unstable world amassed with suffering, pain, sickness, and ageing (see 4), an overall Buddhist 'coping strategy' for contingency might be discernable (similar, i.e. the functional equivalent, to "God", which according to Luhmann, is the formula of contingency for the Christian tradition). Of central importance in this context is the concept of *karma* (rebirth according to the moral quality of action). Below, I will discuss if this concept could—at least for some Buddhist traditions—be seen as a Buddhist formula for 'contingency reduction'.

As a tool to analyze where and how moral expectations or ethical guidelines of religious scholars compete with—or substantially contradict—liberal positions in the

[3] Probably it has been formulated best by the philosopher Richard Rorty: "The process of de-divinization which I described [. . .] would, ideally, culminate in our no longer being able to see any use for the notion that finite, mortal, contingently existing human beings might derive the meanings of their lives from anything except other finite, mortal, contingently existing human beings". And his antidote to this: "We are doomed to spend our conscious lives trying to escape from contingency rather than [. . .] acknowledging and appropriating contingency" [22, p 28].

biomedical and bioethical field, I suggest the application of the categories of 'salvetive' (from the Latin *salveo*, "to heal") and 'salvative' (from Latin *salvo*, "to rescue", "to liberate") dimensions. Salvetive dimensions and narrations, on the one hand, encompass all those practices and moral action-guides that do not interfere with the essential ethical and soteriological teachings of the respective religious tradition.[4] Salvative dimensions, on the other hand, are for example structured by central teachings how to achieve religious goals. Normally, they encompass the highest normative expectations and are connected to strong moral feelings. The scope of both the salvetive and the salvative dimension may vary *between* and *within* specific religious traditions. Moreover, even research practices and expectations of at least some biomedical actors may be described as salvative.

Certainly, predictions concerning one's remaining life span, one's future health conditions, cognitive abilities or reproductive capabilities, are not only expectations in regard to the 'length' and 'quality' of life, but affect existential dimensions in regard to the meaning of 'life' as well. Conceptualized from a religious point of view, scientifically based predictions of a person's limited life-span, etc., may belong more to the salvetive dimension, according to religious specialists of one tradition, whereas specialists of other traditions will see these predictions as an 'interference' with the salvative sphere. In my opinion, those (strands in) religious traditions that encompass (combine, or have certain elements of): (a) a strong distinction between body and soul or immanence and transcendence, and (b) do not 'moralize' illness as 'religious fate', and (c) do not stick to a strict catalogue of sharply defined moral action-guides, have less difficulty to adapt to biomedical diagnostics, predictions and practices.

But how does the Buddhist 'worldview' of *karma* fit into this scheme? To take a very general point of view (which is always a dangerous enterprise), Asian religious traditions of Buddhism, Confucianism, Daoism, and the Hindu traditions seem to find certain commonalities in a quite broadly shared naturalism (or even, a perspective of some kind of 'natural law'). There are no absolute distinctions between a transcendent sphere of God or the natural and the artificial. Human life is, quite often, intertwined with a greater natural order, which is neither totally contingent nor created according to some super-human being.

> "Instead of setting the human life-world apart from nature, there is a general tendency to see it as a part of nature and integrated in the natural order. Polar complementarity and pure immanence instead of a dichotomy between the individual and culture or society are frequently taken to provide ideal-typical paradigms of such alternative models of rationality and ethics" [2, p 279].

An illustrative example of such an Asian view of disease and 'futile treatment', which not only takes into account the biological strands but also a complex system of interpreting contingency (in the salvative dimension), can be seen in the Buddhist theory of *karma*.

---

[4] To be more precise, we may analyze certain schools or teachings of an identifiable subgroup of adherents, not 'religions' as such.

As is well known, rebirth according to the 'quality' of good, bad, or neutral deeds serves in the Buddhist tradition (but also the Hindu and Jain traditions of India) as a framework to explain the current status quo of a living being. There are two different types of *karma*—associated with negative deeds and positive deeds. More specifically, *karma* is classified by moral quality as good or wholesome (Sanskrit *kushala*), unwholesome (*akushala*), and indeterminate (*avyâkrta*).[5] Unwholesome acts result in unhappy rebirth (a list of 'ten evil acts' is organized in terms of bodily, vocal, and mental deeds: taking life, taking what is not given, sexual misconduct, false speech, etc.). Good or 'skilful' acts result in propitious rebirth. Indeterminate acts do not have a karmic result. This theory is the framework in which Buddhists evaluate the meaningfulness of deeds even in the sphere of medical ethics (see 8; compare with 11). In this worldview, human beings are the arbitrators of their own actions and therefore highly dependent on their 'moral' qualities. This concept may be called 'perpetrator-centred' (see 12, p 202), since every individual will experience the karmic forces of his deeds in the future, in contrast to 'victim-centred' approaches (e.g. the assumption of 'human dignity').

From a Buddhist perspective, 'persons' are seen to be in part contingent—dependent upon their constituent parts, their environment, and so on—but, simultaneously, they exert free moral agency (see 19, p 307). However, from early on, the theory of *karma* has not been the sole and single means to reduce the contingency of one's (medical) fate. The following quotation from a famous text of the first century BC, *The Questions of King Milinda* [21], may illustrate this point. There, a Buddhist monk explains:

> "'It is not all suffering that has its root in Karma. There are eight causes by which sufferings arise, by which many beings suffer pain. [. . .]. And therein whosoever maintains that it is Karma that injures beings, and besides it there is no other reason for pain, his proposition is false. [. . .] If [. . .] all diseases were really derived from Karma then there would be no characteristic marks by which they could be distinguished one from the other. When the wind is disturbed, it is so in one or other of ten ways—by cold, or by heat, or by hunger, [. . .], or by medical treatment, or as the result of Karma. Of these ten, nine do not act in a past life or in a future life, but in one's present existence. Therefore it is not right to say that all pain is due to Karma. [. . .] And there is the act that has Karma as its fruit, and the pain so brought about arising from the act done. So what arises as the fruit of Karma is much less than that which arises from other causes. And the ignorant go too far when they say that every pain is produced as the fruit of Karma. No one without a Buddha's insight can fix the extent of the action of Karma'" (translation by Rhys Davids;12, pp 191–192).

Interestingly, this ancient text counts on some 'naturalistic' (and contingent) factors in the explanation of pain, illness, and suffering, and reduces the 'religious' impact to just one factor among others. Furthermore, the ordinary individual's *karma* and its influence in the future cannot be known;[6] therefore, it should not be of use

---

[5] For this publication, a simplified transcription of Sanskrit has been chosen.
[6] According to the Thai Buddhist bioethicist Pinit Ratanakul, the *karma*-interpretation can, however, be useful as a 'contingency formula' in regard to past and present: "A disease", he explains on the one hand, "with a kammic [karmic, J.S.] cause cannot be cured until that kammic result is exhausted" [19, p 309]; on the other hand, medical treatment "does not interefere with the workings of the individual *kamma* but reduces its severity" [19, p 310].

for predictions. This largely shared normative 'academic' opinion, however, is not always relevant for Buddhists, e.g. the modern Tibetan Mahāyāna or South-Asian Theravāda traditions. In these traditions, astrological practices are frequently used to acquire some kind of knowledge—there are even 'signs' forecasting a person's 'medical fate'. The anthropologist Bob Simpson has done extensive research on the interface between local belief- and value-systems and genetic and reproductive technologies in Sri Lanka, and illustrates how these traditional views contribute to the perception of predictive biomedicine:

> "Prenatal diagnostic testing yields a [. . .] dangerous knowledge. Once known, the intimations of the future that are found in chromosomes and genes cannot be un-known and, furthermore, once known give rise to some of the most challenging ethical dilemmas imaginable. The widespread belief, particularly among Buddhists and evidenced in beliefs in karmic consequences and the popularity of astrology, that the future can be known and anticipated through signs that are available in the present, is crucial in understanding the form that these dilemmas take. Genes, as a form of karmic inscription revealed by diagnostic testing, are likely to be given a particular place in attempts to make sense of misfortune" [29, p 40].

'Knowing the Fate'? Tibetan Medical Scriptures on 'Refusing Treatment' of Terminally Ill

The relevance of the assumed 'point of no return' for the question of how medical fate is conceptualized in Asian traditions can be shown by an early example from the pre-modern Tibetan Buddhist tradition. The *Four Tantras* (Tib. *rGyud bzhi*), the standard handbook of Tibetan Medicine written in the 14th century, declares that the necessity to prolong life is not in every case the foremost duty of the healer-physician. As a regulative principle, a healer-physician should learn to distinguish fatal illnesses which exclude further treatment. More precisely, in chapter 26 of the *Explanation-book* (Tib. *bzhad rgyud*) of the rGyud bzhi with the title *Four Parameter of Accepting or Refusing Treatment of Patients* the following explanation is given: "There are four diagnostic criteria for accepting or declining to accept [a patient] according to whether he or she is (1) easy, or (2) difficult to cure, (3) barely treatable, or (4) to be refrained from accepting" (translation by Clark; [3, p 203]). In the latter category, there are two groups of patients: those for whom a treatment exists, and those for whom no therapy is available. An important indicator for non-acceptance—even though treatment is available—is the following: "if his lifespan is exhausted" [3, p 204]. In regard to the group which are, moreover, beyond the point where treatment would be possible, the rGyud bzhi states: "With respect to the type of patient who is not to be accepted in the view of the absence of a means of treatment, if he is beyond hope, bears the signs of death, or if he is seized by (any) of the nine fatal diseases [the doctor] should not accept him" [3, p 204]. In other words, those who irreversibly follow the course of death shall not be treated—even if it would be possible to prolong their life to a certain extent. In our terminology, this means treatment should be seized if the 'point of no return (a)' is reached. Patients belonging to the second group ('absence of treatment') might be conceptualized as having reached the 'point of no return (b)' in the more narrow sense.

Additionally, another chapter of this medical handbook is devoted to an extensive explanation of the *Signs of Death* (see 25, pp 36–40). A person's medical fate may be detected by some types of distant omens, such as (1) messengers (certain people arriving in certain manners), (2) dream omens, and (3) certain ways of malfunctioning of the body. Those 'imminent signs of death' include the following observable, bodily signs:

"[L]oss of blood from the nine orifices without having been affected by poison or weapons; immediately forgetting what has been said; retraction of the penis with the scrotum left hanging down or vice versa; the onset of an unusual sound when clearing the throat [. . .], no appearance of light when one presses one's eyes; having a fixed stare like a rabbit [etc.]" [3, pp 71–72].

Why has it been of such an importance for Tibetan healer-physicians of the 14th century—and one finds similar chapters in medical texts of the Indian ayurvedic as well as the early Chinese tradition—to know the signs of an imminent death? And why should a doctor not try to treat those people, who shouldn't be accepted as patients? One explanation is given in text: because trying to treat non-curable diseases could damage not only the reputation of an individual doctor but of medicine as such.

Yet, another interpretation seems to be possible, too: doctors should not interfere with the salvative dimension, the ('medical') fate of a person beyond the 'point of no return', because he or she is already belonging in part to another realm. It is much more important for the patient to mentally prepare the next rebirth, since, according to the Buddhist view, the personal mental attitude is very important for this process.[7] A good death is characterized by an attitude of mental tranquillity, the absence of fear, and other disturbing attitudes such as hate, greed, or attachment to life—and being able to realize such a mental state while dying will result in a better rebirth as well.[8] Being able to experience a 'good death' is, as Karma Lekshe Tsomo points out, a matter of practice on a long-term, regular basis:

"Clinging to the body creates tremendous tension that actually increases physical as well as mental pain. Meditation on impermanence relaxes the preconceptions of the mind and

---

[7] In addition, a more 'deceptive' strategy (allegedly not influenced by Buddhist principles), has been observed in Japan. Gerhold Becker summarizes: "It seems a common characteristic of medical practice in [. . .] East Asia that disclosure of diagnosis and prognosis is likely to be modified according to the family's opinion. The family, in cooperation with the physician, decides how much information should be shared with the patient about his or her health conditions or the prospects of disease. If the diagnosis concerns terminal illness, the virtue of humaneness or benevolence would demand to keep such disturbing news hidden from the patient as long as possible" [2, p 284].

[8] "The moment of death is a great opportunity for realization. Coming face-to-face with death and impermanence, suffering, and the immanent dissolution of the illusory self are all opportunities for gaining insight into these basic Buddhist truths. Sufferings can be understood as the result of one's own actions in the past, rather than some inexplicable injustice. Through the experience of suffering of illness and approaching death, this negative karma is expiated and it is possible to achieve profound realizations of suffering, impermanence, karma, and much else" [11, p 188].

expectations of one's own physical continuity, which results in a feeling of greater ease and wellbeing" (from 11, p 188; compare with 32, pp 71–73).

Additionally, this example may show how medical and religious specialists compete when it comes to essential issues and soteriological teachings of a respective religious tradition; in this example, the healer-physician is called not to interfere in the final phase of life that is considered by religious specialists of 'salvational' importance.[9] This attitude of non-interference can, moreover, be linked to the workings of *karma*. In the context of euthanasia (which is not allowable for many Buddhist ethicists), Suwanda Sugunasiri points out: "If a handicap or chronic illness is then a 'working off' of one's karma, then euthanasia may be, in fact, an unkind intervention. For it might mean that the sentient being might need one or more births to complete the 'unfinished business'" [32, p 7].

To conclude, the view of *karma*, although important, is not a single overall coping strategy of contingency. Referring to the distinctions above, I would describe *karma* as a contingency formula in the salvetive dimension (and, moreover, predominantly used from a third-person perspective), whereas the salvative contingency formula is of the 'first-person perspective' and is the Buddhist realization of the impermanence, emptiness, and selflessness[10] of all phenomena, i.e. to give up 'clinging' (see 19, pp 95–296).

Predictive Medicine: Some Views of Buddhist Specialists

How do Buddhist ethicists respond to the new practices of predictive medicine, such as prenatal genetic diagnosis, pre-implantation diagnosis, or carrier testing? First, I assume that in the case of prenatal diagnostics the hermeneutics of the 'point of no return' might not be of great value because the predictions do not pertain to persons and their immediate prospective future from a 'first-person perspective'. In these cases, the life of a person is not (yet) conceptualized by the person concerned but by others. Religious strategies for how to cope with predictions of suffering or a limited lifespan, etc. of a yet unborn child, are, therefore, asymmetrical, because parents and other people are able to choose, whereas they are, at the same time, not themselves endangered by life-threatening options (e.g. in the case of abortion). This is, however, not to say that the choices for predictive testing and the options that can be chosen

---

[9] "If all the activities run in biomedical research are mostly just for 'you will have more time to live in this world through this,' the question is: is it rational to devote our energy just to have the 'more time?' [. . .T]his [. . .] is not necessary in the view of Buddhism. However, biomedical research has some potential that Buddhism might agree with. It is the potential to reduce bodily pain caused by disease [. . .]. Having no pain is included in the meaning of well-being in Buddhism, but to have more time is not. So, what to be known is: how to reduce pain or abolish sickness; and what not necessary to know is: how to have more time to live in the world" [16, p 277].

[10] I can only mention the Buddhist 'No-self'-theory as a blueprint of 'weak person'-approaches (see 6, pp 409–411).

thereafter are not 'existential' for those concerned. More precisely, it can be described as a two-fold decision: parents decide on the worthiness of predictive information regarding the offspring's health as well as empower themselves regarding decisions on possible actions.

Given these circumstances, the situation of predictive testing seems to encompass—in direct comparison to aetiopathological predictions—more aspects of non-religious or 'non-salvative' quality, such as economic factors (see 26, 29). Yet, normative expectations in classical Buddhist texts do exert a certain influence on current attitudes. First, Buddhist specialists demand a general attitude of 'acceptance of *karma*' (but not in a fatalistic way) and 'disenchantment' in case of bodily deficiencies. They put stress on the fact that a life is always worth living (particularly if the Buddhist salvative practices can be carried out or mental attitudes trained by the respective individual). These abilities—to overcome suffering—are rooted in the individual, and can only be accomplished by the individual. Thus, the 'third person perspective' of parents, in the case of some kind of predictive 'positive testing', gets relieved from full responsibility. Simpson, who has observed differences between attitudes by Christian or Buddhist individuals in Sri Lanka in his empirical studies, confirms this:

> "Some parents talked of children [. . .] by derogatory terms such as 'mongol' [. . .] (*mongol kiyanava* [. . .]). For [. . .] Buddhists there is usually the added burden of feeling that, in ways that they could never possibly know, parents themselves have contributed to their misfortune (*avasenava*) with the physical appearance of the child seen as public and incontrovertible evidence of a sin committed in a previous life [. . .]. Whereas Christian parents of children with Down's syndrome [. . .] have tended to see their circumstance as a special challenge or test from God, Buddhists, on the contrary, are more passive in their adversity, accepting the child as the working through of an all-embracing law of karma [. . .]. For some parents, the consequences of their actions were thought to happen in a quite direct fashion [. . .]. For others, karma was thought of in a far more nebulous fashion" [29, p 36].

This opinion in regard to prenatal diagnosis of Down's syndrome has been reported by Ratanakul as well: "Thai women will rarely abort it, for they believe that, for the benefit of the foetus, it is better to let its bad karmic effect exhaust itself in the present even if a still-born child is the result" [17, p 59]. This attitude is closely connected to the general Buddhist ethical principle of non-harming sentient beings; abortion, therefore, is evaluated by many Buddhists specialists as impermissible—even in the case of serious defections. As in other traditions, however, Buddhist lay people may evaluate these matters differently by taking into account not only ethical principles but also financial aspects, etc.

Lastly, regarding the feasibility of predictive diagnosis of minor defects in adults, Buddhist ethicists seem to have no clear stance. This question touches on the difficult issue if the knowledge of certain possible constrictions or impairments will imply additional suffering or rather enable the affected individual to practice Buddhist 'salvative coping'.

An important aspect in the Buddhist approach consists of the evaluation of a certain predictive diagnosis: does it in consequence imply mental or psychological harm? Mental harm of the affected individual can indeed be enlarged by (genetic) "discrimination or stigmatization" [6, pp 409–411]. Although the fact that Buddhist ethical specialists point to the conception of the conventional existence of persons (being ultimately empty), they advise all parties (parents and physicians) to evaluate their actions and deeds in respect to the criterion if these actions will bring forth—as a direct consequence—future harm.

Although I mainly focused on Buddhist opinions on prediction in situations of medical futility and could only take a short look on prediction in prenatal diagnostics, I hope that some general strands of Buddhist attitudes toward predictive medicine could be characterized. Whether the hermeneutics of the 'point of no return' and the distinction between 'salvetive' and 'salvative' dimensions are of general use in the contexts of biomedicine and religion(s) is yet to be proven.

Questions and Answers

Q. [*Manuel Battegay*]: How strongly does the concept of 'rebirth' influence the attitude towards medicine? Is it really influencing almost all fields, as you allude?

A. [*Schlieter*]: Well, I think 'rebirth' is actually not a particularly influential aspect, at least not explicitly. If you look at, for example, the Journal of Biomedical Ethics in India, you very rarely see allusions to Indian religious traditions. This holds true for certain Japanese journals as well. Even if religious tradition is the backbone of self-understanding of some individuals—it is not part of the academic discourse on bioethics, which is even more secular than in Europe; they very often present themselves as not using religious arguments.

Q. [*Klaus Lindpaintner*]: As Asian societies are being transformed by modern medicine and as we understand more and know more in advance, is the role of karma receding in these societies? […] Are there going to be fourteen or twenty-one additional causes of illnesses and death other than karma?

A. [*Schlieter*]: This is a very interesting question. A few bioethicists really argue for an identification of the DNA with karma, but this poses several problems regarding procedure. For example, with cloning procedures: If several genetically identical twins would be produced, this would not accord with the idea of an individual karma. There is no collective karma—it has to be an individual karma because it is related to certain acts in former lives. In a way, I see the biomedical advances and explanations as a secularizing force and I find the discourse on karma to be receding or becoming a more metaphorical discourse in which religious sources are taken less literally.

Q. [*Dieter Birnbacher*]: One interesting question concerning the relation of medicine to religion is: To what extent has traditional religion achieved a frame of consciousness, which has survived the 'end of religion'. This may be the case in our [Western] civilization. I think this may also be the case in Asian societies like

Japan, for example. Here we have, among the younger people, a resistance against the Japanese traditions and in favor of more patient autonomy and more open and truthful communication, even in final conditions. This is completely alien to Japanese traditions, as you showed. On the other hand, we have this deep resistance against the brain death criterion, which seems to be so deeply ingrained in the culture itself that it is resistant to any influence by modern biomedicine.

A. [*Schlieter*]: The brain death discussion in Japan is a very good example. Since 1997, there is a law in Japan, which allows patients to choose if they want to be declared dead by the traditional criteria or by the Harvard criteria of brain death. This is quite interesting because it means people can decide how they want to be declared dead. And it has implications: Those who opt for the Harvard criteria are, very often, also those who vote for organ donation, whereas the application of the more strict Japanese criteria exclude the further use of certain organs. This is quite an interesting aspect. On the other hand, it is very difficult for research in religion to capture implicit traditional attitudes, which are stored in the cultural memory and which are affected and brought into play in many different ways: for example, in cartoons or certain mangas, which depict Japanese traditions. In these ways, 'traditional' information may reach the younger generation too, if not only through the study of the traditional sources. It is really very difficult to work out how traditional attitudes work and influence present discourses.

References

1 Sleeboom-Faulkner M (ed): Frameworks of Choice: Predictive and Genetic Testing in Asia. Amsterdam, Amsterdam University Press, 2010.

2 Schlieter J: Bioethik, Religion und Kultur aus komparativer Sicht: Zur Bedeutung und Methodik einer neuen Fragestellung. Polylog 2005;13:7–14.

3 Becker GK: Normative relations: east Asian perspectives on biomedicine and bioethics; in Düwell M, Rehmann-Sutter C, Mieth D (eds): Life Nature Contingency. Dordrecht, Kluwer/Springer, 2008, 273–288.

4 Keown D: Buddhism and Human Rights. Richmond, Curzon Press, 1998, pp 221–222.

5 Mieth D: Die Krise des Fortschritts und die vergessene Endlichkeit des Menschen; in Mieth D (ed.): Moral und Erfahrung—Grundlagen einer theologisch-ethischen Hermeneutik. Freiburg, Herder, 1999, 193–210.

6 Mieth D: Science, religion, and contingency; in Rehmann-Sutter C, Düwell M, Mieth D (eds), Bioethics in Cultural Contexts. Reflections on Methods and Finitude. Berlin, Springer, 2006, 53–69.

7 Miyata H, Tachimori H, et al: Disclosure of cancer diagnosis and prognosis: a survey of the general public's attitudes toward doctors and family holding discretionary powers. BMC Medical Ethics 2004;5/7 http://ww.biomedcentral.com/1472-6939/5/7 (accessed February 10, 2011).

8 Konrad M: Narrating the New Predictive Genetics–Ethics, Ethnography and Science. Cambridge, Cambridge University Press, 2005.

9 Luhmann N: Soziale Systeme. Frankfurt, Suhrkamp, 1994, 374–375.

10 Hui E: A Confucian ethic of medical futility; in Ruiping F (ed): Confucian Bioethics. Dordrecht, Kluwer, 1999, 127–163.

11 Becker GK: The ethics of prenatal screening and the search for global bioethics; in Julia Tao Lai Po-wah (ed): Cross-Cultural Perspectives on the (Im)Possibility of Global Bioethics. Dordrecht, Kluwer Academic Publishers, 2002, 105–130.

12 Clark B: The Quintessence Tantras of Tibetan Medicine. Ithaca, Snow Lion, 1995.

13 Dash NK (ed): Concept of Suffering in Buddhism. New Delhi, Kaveri Books, 2005.

14 Düwell M, Rehmann-Sutter C, Mieth D (eds): Life Nature Contingency. Dordrecht, Kluwer/Springer, 2008.

15 Hongladarom S: Privacy, the individual and genetic information: a Buddhist perspective. Bioethics 2009;23:403–412.

16 Lekshe Tsomo K: Into the Jaws of Yama: Buddhism, Bioethics, and Death. Albany, State University of New York Press, 2006.

17 Mettanando B: Buddhist ethics in the practice of medicine; in Wei-hsun Fu C, Wawrytko SA (eds): Buddhist Ethics and Modern Society. New York, Greenwood Press, 1991, 195–213.

18 Promta S: What to be known and what to be unknown. The Chulalongkorn Journal of Buddhist Studies 2006;5:365–377.

19 Ratanakul P: A survey of Thai Buddhist attitudes towards science and genetics; in Fujiki N, Macer DRJ (eds): Intractable Neurological Disorders, Human Genome Research and Society. Christchurch, Eubios Ethics Institute, 1994, 199–202.

20 Ratanakul P: Socio-medical aspects of abortion in Thailand; in Keown D (ed): Buddhism and Abortion. Basingstoke, McMillan, 1998, 53–65.

21 Ratanakul P: Bioethics and Buddhism. Bangkok, Mahidol, 2004.

22 Rehmann-Sutter C, Düwell M, Mieth D (eds): Bioethics in Cultural Contexts. Reflections on Methods and Finitude. Berlin, Springer, 2006.

23 Rhys Davids TW: The Questions of King Milinda (translation). Oxford, Clarendon, 1890.

24 Rorty R: Contingency, Irony, and Solidarity. Cambridge, Cambridge University Press, 1989.

25 Schlieter J: Limitless changeability? Buddhist bio-ethics, Habermas, and the question of 'human nature'; in Cauchy V (ed): Philosophy and Culture(s). Proceedings of the XXI World Congress of Philosophy, Istanbul 2003, vol. 7. Ankara, Philosophical Society of Turkey, 2007, 165–171.

26 Schneider J: Vāgīśvarakīrtis Mṛtyuvañcanopadeśa, eine buddhistische Lehrschrift zur Abwehr des Todes. Vienna, Austrian Academy of Sciences Press, 2010.

27 Simpson B: On parrots and thorns: Sri Lankan perspectives on genetics, science and the concept of personhood. Health Care Analysis 2007;15:41–49.

28 Simpson B: Negotiating the Therapeutic Gap: Prenatal Diagnostics and Termination in Sri Lanka. Bioethical Enquiry 2007;5:207–215.

29 Simpson B: We have always been modern: Buddhism, science and the new genetic and reproductive technologies in Sri Lanka. Culture and Religion 2009;10:137–158.

30 Simpson B: A 'therapeutic gap': anthropological perspectives on prenatal diagnostics and termination in Sri Lanka; in Sleeboom-Faulkner M (ed): Predictive Testing and the Social Sciences: Frameworks of Choice in Asia. Amsterdam, Amsterdam University Press, 2010, 27–42.

31 Sleeboom-Faulkner M: Social-science perspectives on bioethics: predictive genetic testing (PGT) in Asia. J Bioeth Inq 2007;4:197–206.

32 Sugunasiri Suwanda HJ: Embryo as Person: Buddhism, Bioethics and Society. Toronto, Nalanda College of Buddhist Studies, 2005.

33 Taniguchi S: A Systematic Structure of Ethics Founded on Causal Conditionary; dissertation, University of Michigan, Ann Arbor, 1996.

Prof. Dr. Jens Schlieter
Science of Religion & Center for Global Studies
University of Berne
Vereinsweg 23
CH–3012 Bern (Switzerland)
Tel. +41 31 631 59 76, E-Mail jens.schlieter@relwi.unibe.ch

Author Index

Subject Index